CKD. Now What?

Living with Kidney Disease plus 190 Amazing Low Salt & CKD Friendly Recipes.

Our Journey into Chronic Kidney Disease and our Essential Steps in avoiding Dialysis and finding Stability.

By Rodney L'Huillier

Preface

When faced with the diagnosis of Chronic Kidney Disease what should you be doing?

What can you be doing to live with the symptoms, stop further decline in kidney function, avoid dialysis, and make life as comfortable and liveable as possible?

Those are the exact questions our family had to take on when my father was faced with this very condition.

And they were questions that we didn't easily find answers for. But we searched, and researched, and implemented.

We successfully found balance and stability, and here within we share all that we discovered.

In this book you will find an intro to some of the new words and jargon you'll be hearing, a layman's intro into the kidney and it's functions, an intro to the tests and stages of CKD, techniques for changing habits, the importance of diet, a collection of CKD friendly recipes, along with a few tips for carers.

Whilst focused on my fathers situation of late stage kidney disease, I believe and hope that it will be useful for everyone who is faced with early or late stage diagnosis.

You will find lots of online resources listed throughout this book, for easy access to those you can find a list of all the references at http://fb.me/ckdnowwhat

Copyright & Disclaimer

This book is not intended to be a substitute for the medical advice of a licensed physician. The reader should consult with their doctor in any matters relating to his/her health.

Facebook: http://fb.me/ckdnowwhat

Table of Contents

Introduction....1
CKD Jargon....11
What is the Kidney and What Does it Do?....18
Chronic Kidney Disease and its Stages....20
Changing Habits and Diet post CKD Diagnosis....24
The Importance of Exercise....35
Our Diet Plan for Living with CKD....39
Tips for Daily Life with CKD....54
Finding Stability with CKD....59
CKD Friendly Recipes....63
- Mains....66
- Sides....97
- Soups....117
- Salads....132
- Salad Dressings....170
- Sauces and Gravies....201
- Marinades, Rubs and Spice Blends....255
- Desserts....271

Introduction

I have to be honest with you, a few years ago I did not even really know exactly where the kidneys were even located. And had even less of an idea about what they did!

But, things were certainly not going to stay that way after a series of events that led me, and the rest of my family on a journey of discovery.

I was in China at the time, and awoke in the middle of the night with a shooting pain in one side of my body, It was intense. I had no idea what was going on and to be honest, not only was I in extreme pain, but also in shock. I was in a foreign country and had no idea what to do. At first, I thought, just relax, it will pass.

After an hour or so I was in a sweat, the pain wasn't going away, it was intensifying and coming in waves. What was going on! The fear factor of being in a foreign country, and by myself, was weighing heavily, and this was something I had never experienced before, and a level of pain that was off-the-charts. Even more worrying was that this pain was coming from inside, at least if it was external I could see the reason and start to rationalise things, but not so.

It was 2 am in the morning when I staggered out onto the street and looked for a taxi. Waving down the first one I saw, jumping in and in a shrieking voice exclaiming: "Yi Yuan, Yi Yuan", which means hospital in Chinese. Thankfully, the driver picked up on the urgency of the situation and hit the gas.

Minutes later I was at the Bao'an Shenzhen Central Hospital. My spoken Chinese was no more than a few words, but I easily conveyed to the nurse the pain and the location. People were pushing trolleys in and out of rooms, while this wasn't a large or new hospital by any means, it was certainly busy for that hour. I got into to see the doctor whose English was about as good as my Chinese but fortunately he was intelligent enough to gather what was going on. Next thing I knew I was getting pain-killer shots in my butt and heading upstairs to get an ultrasound.

And there it was, a whopping 1cm kidney stone trying to push its way out my ureter. The ureter is a tube which connects the kidney to the bladder, it's approx 3-4mm in diameter and that 1 cm stone wasn't exactly going to slide out that hole. Pain explained.

And that's where my journey into learning about the kidney began, but that journey wasn't going to end there, or with just me.

I had several sessions of Shock Wave Lithotripsy which is a kind of electric pulse wave that aimed at the stone with the intention of shattering or fracturing stone into smaller pieces so that it will pass out through the urine. Along with that, I was taking medicine to try and chemically dissolve the stone. It helped, the stone moved a bit and the pain receded. At that time the doctor stated that as long as there is no obstruction and urine can flow, it will be OK to leave it there as for them operating would be difficult due to my weight. I was probably fifteen kilo overweight at that time.

How did I get this stone? There are several types of stones, each with their own causes. Apparently, in my case, it was most likely due to lack of hydration. Other causes are wide-ranging and include family history, high salt diets, digestive diseases, hyperthyroidism, infection and more [1].

According to Kidney Health Australia, the reason for a stone forming in many cases can be unknown [2] and that some 1 in 10 men and 1 in 35 women are likely to suffer from kidney stones in their life.

But, this story is not about me nor is it primarily about kidney stones. It's about Kidney Disease and the journey of my father into what is a life-sapping disease. CKD (Chronic Kidney Disease) is a silent killer in many ways as Kidney Health Australia reveal that less than 10 percent of people with chronic kidney disease are aware they have the condition and that a person can lose up to 90% of their kidney function without experiencing symptoms.

Kidney Health Australia also reports that Kidney-related disease kills more people each year than breast cancer, prostate cancer or even road traffic accidents [3]. That is a chilling fact and makes one wonder why more is not heard about it.

I was still in China at the time my father was flown to the intensive care unit. My father had been in and out of hospital and the specialist for numerous issues and one night at home while getting into bed he simply collapsed. My mother tried to move him but could not and called my brother to come from his home to help. To cut a long story short, next they knew he was in an ambulance and not long after that he was on a flight to an Intensive Care Unit.

He was fighting off organ failure that was later to be discovered caused by an internal infection. It was touch and go, and for hours doctors did everything they could to keep this soul on this planet. And, thankfully, bless them, they won that battle.

After hearing the news, and not knowing how the recovery was going to shape up, or whether there actually would be a recovery, I jumped on a plane and headed home. Arriving at the hospital just a glimpse of my father straight away told me that he was still in a fight for his life.

Even though he had moved out of intensive care he was still being monitored by the hour as the tests were showing that his kidneys were simply not functioning at the required level.

It was an anxious period, not knowing what direction things were going and simply waiting for the next test result to show some sign of hope.

While the doctors and nurses were fantastic at both hospitals, they couldn't tell us the future. As good as science is and with all the modern equipment, training and tests that are available, it's really a day by day thing in these situations.

Fortunately, slowly, day by day, he started showing signs

of bouncing back, not just in the look on his face but also in the test results. Thankfully, his kidneys were showing signs of bouncing back into action.

His days at that point consisted of mostly lying in bed, occasionally lifted to sit in a chair by the window, and visits from us during the afternoons. It took some time for his appetite to come back and it required some coaxing at every meal to get anything in. Likewise with fluids, something the nurses urged more of so as to clear out all the toxins. It was slow going. But day by day he started to improve, the test results were improving, eating more and more, becoming more aware and more responsive. The doctors notified us that he was ready to be moved from high level care and into another ward for rehabilitation.

Even at this point, it was still unsure as to what sort of recovery he was going to make, to be honest it didn't feel like a recovery, it was more like we had just moved out of the danger zone.

During the weeks in the rehabilitation ward, he started to build enough energy to walk again, starting with a 10 meter assisted walk, then a bit more each day until he made it around to a cafe area we would all sit together for an hour or two.

During the time in the rehabilitation ward he was also receiving some physiotherapy to try and get his muscles moving to improve stability, which wasn't easy, as age, arthritis, and the time laying in the hospital were all against him.

Eventually, he was discharged, hardly ready to bounce back into life but, alive, and could finally go home.

At home he had no energy, shortness of breath, often having the urge to vomit, low appetite, frequent toilet visits throughout the day and night, and disturbed sleep. He still had what was described as confusion and some memory issues, which at that stage was attributed to the concoction of medicinal chemicals and disorientating nature of a long stay in hospital. There was a long road ahead.

We were still unsure of what direction things were heading, and what we should be doing, and what others such as specialists and doctors should be doing. There was still a sense of worry, and things were still very much day by day.

My mother was tireless in the care she provided, nursing him through every stage of the day. He needed assistance from morning to night and she did/does a fantastic job of that. My brother and I were merely a support crew.

For my father his daily life at that point consisted of waking around nine, after making numerous trips to the toilet during the night, and spending most of the day seated looking out the front window with regular toilet trips and a bucket was never far away. Some days he looked better than others, but his daily life was a struggle at best, which by default transferred onto my mother.

After sitting by his side all those days in the hospital and waiting for the kidney test results to show a sign of hope, any test results we had post hospital were scrutinized by everyone. And they were not good. Our doctor was distressed by the figures and we were referred to the nephrologist again.

The results indicated that he was teetering on the edge of kidney failure and we were simply playing a waiting game as to whether they would improve, or be needing intervention by dialysis or possibly even transplant. It was an anxious few months, full of trips back and forth from testing labs, doctors, and specialists rooms.

It was at that point we started to understand we were living under a new paradigm, his kidneys were not going to improve in function, we were living with Chronic Kidney

Disease perhaps due to existing decline, age, and obviously the acute shock that his body went through during that near death experience.

What we all wanted is simply to make my fathers and in turn my mother's life as comfortable as possible. I didn't have any expectation of some kind of miracle recovery but simply to make life more comfortable. Going to the toilet 10 times a day, vomiting into a bucket several times a day, being in and out of doctors rooms, and the looming possibility of further decline and the need for dialysis, was simply not my definition of comfortable living for our dad or by extension, mum.

So quite simply, all we really wanted to do, and perhaps all we could do, is to lean everything we could in his favor.

The doctor and specialist's advice is essential, and must be the foundation of any path back to health, but on the home-front, what could we be doing to provide further support? A lot it turns out.

Pouring through the numerous government institutions dedicated to kidney research and public support we found a wealth of information, suggestions for diet and lifestyle along with the comfort to know that this was not a journey we were facing alone.

As stated by the US-based National Kidney Foundation, Chronic Kidney disease is a worldwide health crisis. Not only is it responsible for some 58 million deaths worldwide, it's costing health services and taxpayers billions. The US is expected to spend some $48 billion per year, and in England, chronic kidney disease costs the health services more than breast, lung, colon and skin cancer combined. Australia is expected to spend some 12 billion between now and 2020. Staggering.

In the following chapters, I will walk you through the knowledge we obtained in our efforts to ease the journey with CKD including kidney functions, tests, diet, exercise, changing habits, and a collection of tailored nutritious recipes along with links to numerous key resources.

References

1 http://www.mayoclinic.org/diseases-conditions/kidney-stones/symptoms-causes/dxc-20319562

2 http://kidney.org.au/your-kidneys/detect/kidney-stones/the-causes-437

3 http://kidney.org.au/cms_uploads/docs/kidney-health-australia-kidney-fast-facts-fact-sheet.pdf [PDF]

CKD Jargon

Lets get to know some of the jargon that's going to be coming your way.

Acute kidney injury - is sudden damage to the kidneys.

Albumin - Albumin is a protein made by the liver.

Albumin to Creatinine ratio (ACR) - A urine sample is taken to test the levels of Creatine and Albumin in the urine. ACR is calculated by dividing albumin concentration in milligrams by creatinine concentration in grams which can provide insights into the functioning ability of the kidney.

Anaemia - a shortage of red blood cells in the body with symptoms showing as tiredness, shortness of breath, and paler than usual skin.

Aorta - the largest artery in the body.

Artery - a blood vessel that carries blood from the heart to other organs.

Bladder – the size of a pear, the bladder is a sac storing urine from the kidneys. The bladder allows for urination to be infrequent and voluntary.

Blood Pressure - The heart is like a muscular mechanical pump that, with each beat, squeezes and pushes blood through around your body. The force creates pressure in the arteries which is referred to as systolic blood pressure. The pressure in the arteries when the heart rests between beats is called diastolic blood pressure.

A normal *systolic blood pressure* is below 120 whereas a reading of 140 indicates high blood pressure also known as hypertension. A normal *diastolic blood pressure* is lower than 80 whereas over 90 indicates high blood pressure.

Blood Sugar Levels - a measurement to determine the amount of glucose in your blood.

Catheter – there are numerous types, basically, they are a flexible plastic tube used to enter the interior of the body used to assist in the drainage of urine.

Chronic kidney disease (CKD) - reduced kidney function that lasts for 3 months or more.

Creatinine - a waste product that comes from the normal breakdown of muscle tissue. Everyone has creatinine in their bloodstream and the kidney has a role in filtering out that creatinine waste and discharging it via urine.

Dialysis - treatment which removes toxins, extra salt, and extra fluid from the blood when the kidneys are failing to do so. There are two types of dialysis, haemodialysis, and peritoneal dialysis. Haemodialysis is a process of filtering the blood and is carried out at the hospital or clinic, usually several times per week. Peritoneal dialysis can be done in the home and is a process of introducing a sterile fluid to the abdomen and later draining that fluid. While the fluid is in the abdomen it draws impurities from the blood vessels.

Dietitian/Nutritionist - An expert in food and nutrition.

eGFR/GFR - It is a blood test that can measure the health of your kidneys.

Haemoglobin (Hb) - a substance in red blood cells that carries oxygen around the body. Low Hb levels may indicate anaemia.

Hormones – created by glands in the body, they used to communicate between organs and tissues for physiological regulation and behavioural activities, such as digestion, metabolism, respiration, tissue function, sensory perception, sleep, excretion, lactation, stress, growth and development, movement, reproduction, and mood.

Hyperparathyroidism – Excess production of parathyroid hormone.

Hypertension – High blood pressure.

Hypotension – Low blood pressure.

Oedema – Swelling caused by the accumulation of fluid in the tissue. In can occur in one part of the body or all over depending on the cause. It commonly occurs in the ankles and legs. It can be a symptom of various underlying health conditions.

Polycystic kidney disease - a disorder in which clusters of cysts develop primarily within your kidneys, causing your kidneys to enlarge and lose function over time.

Protein - is an essential nutrient for the human body being one of the building blocks of body tissue, and also serving as a fuel source. Dietary sources of protein include meats, dairy, fish, eggs as well as grains, legumes, and nuts. For some stages of CKD, a nutritionist or doctor may recommend reducing protein intake due to the kidney's inability to filter out protein wastes.

Phosphate - a mineral that helps calcium to strengthen the bones. For some stages of CKD, a nutritionist or doctor may recommend reducing intake of phosphorus via dietary changes.

Potassium - a mineral that helps your body functions yet for some stages of CKD a nutritionist or doctor may recommend reducing intake of potassium via dietary changes.

Reflux nephropathy - A kidney condition caused by urine flowing back into the kidneys due to an obstruction.

Serum creatinine - A measure of how much creatinine is in the blood.

Sodium - a mineral that is present in many natural foods and also increased via the addition of salt. For some stages of CKD especially where blood pressure is a concern, a nutritionist or doctor may recommend reducing intake of salt via dietary changes.

Uraemia - the accumulation of waste products, normally excreted in the urine which can lead to nausea, vomiting, tiredness, and problems with concentration.

Urea - A waste product of the breakdown of protein in

the liver which is then removed from the bloodstream via the kidney.

Ureter - the tube by which urine passes from the kidney to the bladder

Urethra - the tube by which urine is passed out of the body from the bladder

UTI - Urinary tract infections

Nephron – the functioning unit of the kidney, with each kidney containing over a million.

What is the Kidney and What Does it Do?

As I am sure you know, there is not just one, there are two kidneys. These bean-shaped organs are located on either side of the spine towards the bottom of the rib cage. Why two? So vital is their function that we have inbuilt redundancy, if one kidney fails or is damaged in an accident, we can survive with the remaining one. Which reminds me of the many selfless people who donate one of their kidneys to those in desperate need of a transplant. A big shout out to all those wonderful people!

While in simple terms the kidney could be viewed as a waste disposal and recycling unit, it has a wide array of functions and works in concert with other organs throughout the body.

Some of those functions include blood pressure control, hormone secretion, nutrient re-absorption, cleaning the blood, Vitamin D activation, homoeostasis (regulation of PH levels), and regulating salt and water balance.

Each kidney is connected into the bloodstream, with an

inlet and outlet on one side and at the bottom is connected to the bladder via a tube known as the Ureter.

The kidneys inlets are connected to the Aorta, which is the main artery in the body, with the purpose of removing waste and excess fluid from the blood and other tasks as discussed earlier. The filtered blood is then returned to the body via a large vein known as the Inferior Vena Cava. The waste produced in this process, urine, is sent on to the bladder via the Ureter. That waste urine will accumulate in the bladder until it's time to urinate and it passes out of the bladder, and out of the body, via a tube known as the Urethra.

Blood will pass through your kidneys some twelve times a day which translates to the kidneys processing some 200 liters of blood every day. Amazing.

Chronic Kidney Disease and its Stages

According to the American National Kidney Foundation, the causes of Chronic Kidney Disease include Diabetes, High Blood Pressure, Glomerulonephritis, Polycystic Kidney Disease, Lupus, diseases that affect the Immune System, obstructions caused by Kidney Stones, Tumors, an enlarged Prostate (in men), and Urinary Tract Infections.

What's interesting to note is that a reduction in Kidney function can go undetected, and without symptoms, until later stages of CKD. If detected early, there is reportedly a much better chance of slowing or stopping the progression of CKD.

Possible symptoms of kidney disease noticeable in the later stages may be poor appetite, shortness of breath, tiredness, blood in the urine, increased need to urinate at night, insomnia, itching, cramps, feeling sick, headaches, and erectile dysfunction in men. [1]

The Tests

GFR (Glomerular Filtration Rate) or eGFR (estimated Glomerular Filtration Rate) is the go-to test for Kidney function.

It's a blood test that measures the amount of creatine in the blood, creatine comes from muscle tissue activity and when kidney function diminishes so does the ability to filter creatine waste from the blood. A mathematical formula consisting of age, race, and sex is applied to the result to give a GFR/eGFR number which can provide a guide to the state of the kidney.

Albumin to Creatinine ratio (ACR) is a urine test that checks for albumin in your urine. Albumin is a protein that can pass into the urine when the kidneys are damaged and not filtering the blood as they should.

There are several other urine and blood tests the doctor may perform depending on your needs. More about tests here: https://www.healthdirect.gov.au/kidney-function-tests and https://www.kidney.org/atoz/content/understanding-your-lab-values

Another thing to note is that the doctor may not like to make a conclusion until these tests are performed several times and compared over a time period. Your doctor will be trying to establish whether there is a continuing decline, consistency in the figures indicating a new baseline, or a rebound in kidney function post-injury.

The Stages of CKD [2]

Stage 1 with normal or high GFR (GFR > 90 mL/min)
Stage 2 Mild CKD (GFR = 60-89 mL/min)
Stage 3A Moderate CKD (GFR = 45-59 mL/min)
Stage 3B Moderate CKD (GFR = 30-44 mL/min)
Stage 4 Severe CKD (GFR = 15-29 mL/min)
Stage 5 End Stage CKD (GFR <15 mL/min)

Once it's understood as to whether you have a decline in kidney function, and at what stage that may be from there the doctor can suggest a pathway of actions and perhaps even changes to diet which may differ depending on what stage you are at. The doctor may also make referrals to a nephrologist (kidney specialist) and dietician.

Your diet and lifestyle habits are bound to come under close scrutiny along with your cardiovascular condition as a decline in kidney function can lead to serious concerns in this area too. Even if you only have an early stage of CKD, now is the time for taking positive steps for better outcomes.

References

1. Symptoms of Chronic Kidney Disease - http://www.nhs.uk/Conditions/Kidney-disease-chronic/Pages/Symptoms.aspx

2. Stages of Chronic Kidney Disease - https://www.davita.com/kidney-disease/overview/stages-of-kidney-disease

Changing Habits and Diet post CKD Diagnosis

Faced with the new information that you are at some stage of CKD, like we were, it's likely that your doctor and nutritionist are going to be saying it's time to make some changes.

Those changes will likely be different for every person depending on your current lifestyle, your condition, and perhaps even the mindset of your medical practitioners.

Some medical practitioners will place a larger focus on diet and lifestyle than others and that can be for numerous reasons. Whether they are not inclined to believe that nutrition and lifestyle changes can be of benefit, or maybe they resist due to fear of push-back from the patient, maybe they simply don't bother anymore after many failed attempts at giving such advice, or perhaps other reasons. Regardless, any step you can take to try and improve your quality of life is a worthwhile step so, work with your doctor and ask to know everything that you can be doing.

I was excited to know that as part of my father's rehab prior to leaving hospital that he would be visited by a nutritionist. Sadly I was really disappointed to receive a generic flyer on our departure with nothing more than a few sentences singled out by yellow highlighter. I know there is a lot more that can be done and was determined to do so.

So, for your own benefit, you may choose to take the initiative and push your doctor and specialist for quality advice on nutritional and lifestyle practices that are going to benefit your particular situation and suit your needs.

On this journey so far something that keeps hitting me in all the research I do is the fact that when it comes to what's good for us, we are all different. What foods are good for me, might not be good for you and that there is no generic diet that perfectly suits everyone. And CKD provides the perfect example of this, while protein, potassium, and phosphorus are essential for most healthy people it's most certainly advised to reduce consumption in the late stages of CKD.

And there are so many other examples. Bread is such a large part of the western diet, yet, for some, it's quite destructive to their health in many cases due to the gluten. Some people seem to handle bread just fine whereas others it can lead to gut issues, thyroid issues and even, quite dramatically, mental illness according to some studies [1].

Isn't that staggering? One of our daily staples could possibly be causing so much trouble for some of us yet, who talks about these things?

What may be OK for some us is simply not OK for others and that's why consulting a dietician is key. They can assess if there any foods causing immune responses, or foods that may not be suitable for you in your current condition, along with recommending foods which can be of support. And then provide on-going monitoring of those changes, and making adjustments as required, just as your doctor would when prescribing new medicines.

As published in Today's Dietician, several studies have pointed to the wide-ranging benefits of nutrition therapy when it comes to people suffering from CKD and thus make wide-ranging recommendations for assessing if a patient is suffering from malnutrition and methods for reversing such. They strongly recommend patients receiving a nutrition-focused physical exam to determine patients' nutrition status and on-going monitoring [3].

My case is simple, if there is so much value to be gained, it's worth a lot more effort than a simple flyer with some highlighted points.

Continuing on the same theme, a published study reports that among U.S. adults, more than 90 percent of type 2 diabetes, 80 percent of CAD, 70 percent of stroke, and 70 percent of colon cancer are potentially preventable by a combination of non-smoking, avoidance of overweight, moderate physical activity, healthy diet, and moderate alcohol consumption [2]. I think that very observation highlights how removed we have become from the importance of nutrition and lifestyle choices. The suffering caused by these diseases far outweighs any joy derived from the cumulative consumption of tasty snacks, poor lifestyle choices and so on, does it not?

It can be the most bitter pill of all to swallow, the fact that you need to make changes. It's really all about taking responsibility that not only benefits yourself but also those around you.

Start adding up the costs such as spending time in hospital, the cost of doctors visits, the decreased lifestyle, and the toll on family and friends. It's worth making a few changes.

And I really want to push that point home right now, it's family and friends and the community at large who also pay the cost. It's your family that will change their life to help you while you visit the doctor, spend time in hospital and nurse you through to recovery. Sure, they will do that without a second thought, but you have to do your part too.

Now, this is no time to start beating yourself up, nope, you're already going through enough. It's time to pat yourself on the back and say, I can do this, I can be a part of this solution. I can take responsibility.

The benefits of making change can be dramatic, not only to your own quality of life but also to the lives of your family, friends and the community. So, let's embrace change.

I think there is something powerful, and empowering, when you take responsibility for your outcomes and I'm sure that's something you are going to feel proud about, along with family and friends when they see the effort you are making.

Your doctor, your specialist and your nutritionist are going to guide you on the right lifestyle changes for you, and you should push them for all the things that you can do to help improve your odds and lean everything possible in your favor.

Is it going to be easy? No. it won't be. But will it be worth it? Yes. Not only for your health but also for your spirit, you'll be leading the fight for your return to well-being, and that's to be applauded.

Making Change

Awareness

I know for a fact that its a very difficult thing trying to give up old-time favorites, oh boy do I know. When I had a hankering for one type of a food or another, nothing would stop me, even if I had to go drive and get it, regardless of the pantry being full of many healthy food choices. So, what is that drives us to this illogical action? What is that drives food cravings and even worse, binge eating?

As it turns out, eating, along with many other activities, can release a chemical in the brain called dopamine, which is like a feel-good reward [4]. If activated by overeating, or perhaps eating unhealthy comfort foods, then the linkage is created in the brain being do this and feel good. So, it's not only the delicious taste that is desirable, it's also a pleasure hit induced by the brain. And this pleasure hit, relieves stress, for a short time, and makes you relax. And you guessed it, it becomes addictive.

So, what do you do when you feel stressed, or you want to relax? Reach for those unhealthy snacks. The brain in this situation is quite simply rewarding us for the wrong thing in our current set of circumstances.

And that can be a really difficult linkage to become aware of, and to transform into a more healthy habit. But one that we need to to do.

Awareness is the first step. Once we are aware, we can then start transforming and replacing those unhealthy options with healthier choices that will not only make us feel good but also reward us with long-term health and a more comfortable and sustainable existence.

It starts with being mindful, and listening to yourself. When your brain is hammering you with a hankering for a doughnut, or juicy hamburger, it's time to stop, pause, breathe, and understand that linkage that's been created by the release of dopamine, and understand that these foods are simply not good for you in your current situation, and that in the end what your getting is a somewhat of a fake reward.

Healthy rewards and healthy stress management

Once you are aware of your habits and can catch yourself before you dive that hand into the cookie jar, or put that fork into that giant slab juicy steak, or reach out for that salt shaker, it's a case of what to do next. Your doctor and nutritionist should hopefully guide you and work together with you through these challenges.

My belief was that elimination of the bad habit was not the answer, and that habits need to be transformed. You definitely don't want to take away all the things that give you joy and comfort, no no no, we'd go crazy! They just need to be transformed into activities, practices, and methods that also support your recovery and long-term health.

For example, if stress is the trigger for eating something that you shouldn't then look into alternative ways to relieve that stress. For many of us, including myself, the problem was simply not knowing that there is a whole host of options, tools, and methods that can help to relieve stress, bring joy and comfort, without the need for chowing down on a bucket of ice cream to get that feel-good dopamine hit. Knowledge is the key here.

So, it's time to learn a few new tricks and put some tools in your toolbox. We are all different and we all have our own likes and dislikes, so it's about finding the methods and activities that are going to suit you and your situation.

Again this is something to work on with your doctor and specialists. I will suggest a few generic resources just to get the mind ticking.

6 Steps to Changing Bad Eating Habits - http://www.webmd.com/diet/obesity/features/6-steps-to-changing-bad-eating-habits#1

How to Change a Habit for Good - https://www.mindful.org/how-to-change-a-habit-for-good/

7 Steps to Changing a Bad Habit - https://psychcentral.com/lib/7-steps-to-changing-a-bad-habit/

Step by Step

If a drastic change is required it can seem like being confronted with an impassable mountain. And it can be stressful.

But it's like anything in life, and every journey to a destination is a series of steps that begins with the first. And that's really the secret here, step by step. When faced with something that seems impossible to handle as a whole, break into small pieces and tackle it step by step. And with each step, congratulate yourself, as each step made is a step closer and your making that mountain shrink before your very eyes! So, step by step.

Don't beat yourself up

if you fall off, just get back on. It's that simple. If you fall to temptation and snacked on something you shouldn't have, don't beat yourself up, just commit to getting back on track. If it keeps happening then you may need to make a more succinct change, like not stocking those items in your pantry or not walking past that cake shop. But always remember, if you get off track, don't beat yourself up and make yourself give in, no, no, no, just dust yourself off, recommit to your health goals, and get back on track. Easy as that.

References:

1. Bread and Other Edible Agents of Mental Disease - https://www.ncbi.nlm.nih.gov/pmc/articles/PMC4809873/

2. Prevention of Chronic Disease by Means of Diet and Lifestyle Changes - https://www.ncbi.nlm.nih.gov/books/NBK11795/

3. Assessing Nutrition in Patients With Chronic Kidney Disease - http://www.todaysdietitian.com/pdf/courses/ThompsonCKD.pdf

4. Addicted to Fat: Overeating May Alter the Brain as Much as Hard Drugs - https://www.scientificamerican.com/article/addicted-to-fat-eating/

The Importance of Exercise

The National Kidney Foundation (USA) states the benefits of exercise [1] as such

- Improved muscle physical functioning

- Better blood pressure control

- Improved muscle strength

- Lowered level of blood fats (cholesterol and triglycerides)

- Better sleep

- Better control of body weight

I don't really think anyone needs to be sold on the benefits of increased fitness. For some people, it's already very much a part of their life whether they go to the gym on a regular basis, play sport, yoga, go for walks of a morning or night and so on. For others, it may not be a part of their life at all, and that may be hindering their quality of life.

Before starting any exercise plan, you must talk with your doctor. Get their assessment of what is suitable for you and your condition and even enlist the services of a physiotherapist to help develop a plan tailored to your needs and desired outcome.

For my father, it was a struggle, his days of boxing, football, gym, and hard-yakka were a very distant memory. He was a guy who very much deserved to put his feet up and that's something he was very determined to achieve. Rightly so, with all that was going on in his body, there was little energy or enthusiasm for any kind of activity, on top of that there was the pain of arthritis.

Arthritis is such a terrible thing, one of those diseases that's hidden from view, only the person with it knows how much pain it's delivering. If your leg was in plaster everyone would have an instant visual verification of yes, that person is in difficulty, not so with arthritis and many other diseases for that matter.

Taking all those things into account we coaxed him into light exercises as recommended by the physician and later the doctor also referred him to a physiotherapist. This was a great move and not only was another excuse for him to get out of the house but also get moving.

And moving is what it's all about. If you're starting from zero, then just simply moving is a great place to start. Moving the arms, moving the legs, anything is going to help and little steps in the right direction will lead to bigger and bigger steps.

I cant speak here as to what exercise you should be doing, that depends on your status and condition and the advice of your doctor/physiotherapist. We are all different.

I can only suggest that it is an essential part of the solution and another key to living a comfortable life with CKD. Discuss it with your doctor and push for a referral to a physiotherapist to get you on track with an exercise plan to suit you.

And here's the kicker, for those that cringe at the thought of exercise and activity, you might be in for a big surprise! It's fun! Really.

In my own personal journey I was a person who procrastinated about doing exercise in a big way, but after setting a routine and sticking to it for no more than a few weeks something amazing happened. I went from loathing the thought of doing exercise to craving it. I started off slowly, but kept to a regular schedule and slowly began doing more and more, and I was doing more and more not because I had to but because I wanted to.

Something else happened too, I was feeling good after doing exercise not only from the benefits of doing exercise but also from the fact that I had overcome my procrastination and was moving forward in a positive way. I feel that it has a big physiological effect and that positivity transforms into hope and the ability to overcome other challenges. I cannot recommend it enough. Just do it!

A resource that I found to be incredibly useful personally is BodyBuilding.com, whilst the name conjures images of Schwarzenegger types lifting insane amounts of weights, it is actually very much a place for everyone, with free programs for all levels, and home to countless people who have transformed themselves for various reasons.

1. Staying Fit with Kidney Disease - https://www.kidney.org/atoz/content/stayfit

2. Health and fitness - A range of exercise and activity guides for all age groups - http://www.nhs.uk/livewell/fitness/Pages/Fitnesshome.aspx

3. How to start exercising if you're out of shape - https://www.health.harvard.edu/staying-healthy/how-to-start-exercising-if-youre-out-of-shape-

Our Diet Plan for Living with CKD

When facing a chronic illness I believe one of the most important things to do in tandem with seeing your doctor is to also consult a trained nutritionist. In particular, a Renal Dietician when you are suffering kidney disease. This is certainly something recommended by Kidney Health Australia [1] and the importance of diet in dealing with kidney disease is something you can't escape with every global institution dedicating realms of information to the topic.

For some people, adopting a nutrition based lifestyle and making adjustments to new requirements is not such a big deal although, it can be a huge challenge for others. Especially the older you are, changing habits is no simple task.

I think this is a point the doctors were much more aware of then me. When diet was mentioned, it seemed to be a background issue and being happy and enjoying the time seemed to have greater importance. I can certainly understand that thinking, I really can. But is that what happiness is nowadays? A fatty, salty feast followed by a cream bun?

If eating certain foods are diminishing the overall quality of life why would you eat them? It's like saying it's OK to smoke because you enjoy it or it's OK to take drugs if it makes you happy. The short-term benefit is not worth the long-term cost.

I am not, nor proclaim to be a medical expert, but from my research about what the kidney does, and the effect of its diminishing role when suffering from kidney disease, it just seems so important to be tailoring a diet specific to one's needs. The kidney simply can't process things like a healthy person would particularly in the late stages if CKD.

Like I mentioned before, going to hospital, visiting doctors, vomiting into buckets, and spraying the toilet bowl every two hours simply isn't 'quality of life'. These are the obvious visible symptoms, then there's things going on that we don't see, if the Kidney isn't filtering as it should, any excess toxins are remaining in the blood which can only have long-term negative effects.

So again, why not stack everything in your favor? If you have to cut salt, just cut it. If you have to cut bread, just cut it. If you can make changes to the diet that improve and support the digestive process, then do it.

The takeaway here is to work positively with a dietician, and your relationship with them could be just as important as that with your doctor.

For us, the nutritional advice received from the hospital on departure was sadly a vague and generic flyer. Living with my mum and dad and taking on the role of meals while my mother was pretty much the 24/7 nurse on duty, I felt it critical to know what's good, and what's not, and what can we be doing better. Anything that's going to improve the quality of life.

Fortunately, there is a wide array of information published by credible sources and I will share those here.

Kidney Health Australia - http://kidney.org.au
Da Vita - https://www.davita.com
American Association of Kidney Patients - https://aakp.org
Kidney Patient Guide - http://www.kidneypatientguide.org.uk
Kidney Research UK - https://www.kidneyresearchuk.org
The National Institute of Diabetes and Digestive and Kidney Diseases

Health Information Center - https://www.niddk.nih.gov/

A key takeaway from those sites is the fact that as the kidney progresses into later stages of CKD it's ability to filter out protein waste and minerals declines. Some of the effects include [2]:

As discussed in an earlier chapter, a key role of the kidney is to regulate salt and fluids in the bloodstream. Poor regulation of salt and fluids can lead to excess fluids collecting in the lungs, swelling, breathing difficulties and strain on the heart.

With declining function the kidney can also lose its ability to regulate potassium, an essential nutrient yet in excess can affect muscle function and affect the heart.

The kidney also removes waste products left over from the breakdown of proteins, if unfiltered they are like poison to the body leading to feelings of nausea and fatigue.

The kidney also releases vital hormones which help regulate blood pressure and help the bone marrow produce red blood cells. A low production of red blood cells is a cause of Anemia.

The kidney also produces Vitamin D which assists calcium absorption and without it, bone disease can be the end result.

Alongside my mother and brother, I first hand witnessed many of these effects, and it's painful watching someone vomit into a bucket, and to have no energy, to have confusion, and to have the look that 'the day is near'. If there's a possible path away from that, I'm sure I am going to help my father get it.

My thinking was simple, do as much as possible to take the load of the kidney, boost nutrition as much as possible and keep the fluid intake up to help clear away toxins as much as possible. At least that was my thinking, no, not looking for a miracle cure, just some quality of life.

The basics of that plan were simple enough and guided by the advice drawn from researching the leading literature and research studies from the key kidney institutions and medical institutes, together with the nephrologists advice, which were:

- Limit salt intake
- Limit protein and portion control for meat servings
- Decrease and limit the foods that are high in potassium

and phosphorus

- Increase nutrient intake from beneficial foods
- Introduce probiotic foods
- Aim for 1-1.5 liters of fluids
- Keep eating times regular
- Serve the last major meal no later than 6.30

Why the last meal before 6.30? Recent studies have suggested that the late night eating had poor consequences for blood pressure [3] and also as there seems to be much support for the fact that the digestive process slows during the night.

Which led me to consider another point which is the effect of poor digestive health for people with CKD? And apparently, I am not the only one. Fabiola Martín del Campo, a researcher at the University of Guadalajara in Mexico recently had a study published by the National Kidney Foundation's Journal of Renal Nutrition [4] which studied the effect of a daily probiotic supplement. The results were positive with reductions in vomiting, heartburn, stomach-ache, and constipation along with improvements in nutrient absorption and reduced inflammation. Actually, the studies into the use of probiotics and nutritional intervention seem to be numerous [5], yet, surprisingly little was ever mentioned about it.

In an article published in the Journal of Preventative Epidemiology by Marzeih Kafeshani Ph.D, the benefits of probiotics and prebiotics were also explored and I quote “It has been detected that toxins produced by gastrointestinal dysbiosis may contribute to CKD progression and complications. Thus the Mediterranean diet, that shifts gut microbial metabolism towards saccharolytic pathway and decreases colonic transit time, with probiotic, prebiotic or symbiotic direction, which may be useful in lessening gut derivative uremic toxins, are ideal and innovative method for CKD patients.”

Medical nutrition therapy (MNT), the microbiome, and gut health is a very hot topic with several major studies in progress such as the Human Microbiome Project - https://www.ncbi.nlm.nih.gov/pmc/articles/PMC3709439/. The microbiome refers to all the microorganisms, such as bacteria, that live within our gut and as scientists are starting to discover, they are playing a large role in our health and well-being, along with perhaps holding solutions to many chronic diseases. Let's hope it can lead us to better information and better outcomes for all.

For my father's diet, I had a big focus on fresh vegetables and adding foods that support gut health such as Greek Yoghurt,

Sauerkraut, and Kombucha. But of course, that also had to be balanced out against the requirements for limiting salt, phosphorus, and potassium due to his progressed stage of CKD. Another point to note with fermented foods is that they must come from the refrigerated section, shelf stored products have been pasteurized and have none of the probiotic benefits that we are looking for.

So that's very much another topic for discussion with your nutritionist and doctor as for what the benefits of assessing gut health and what you may want to introduce or remove, from the diet.

My Fathers Diet

It's difficult to know what foods contain what minerals but fortunately there are many sites that help with this. A fantastic resource for evaluating the properties of different natural foods is http://www.whfoods.com which provides complete breakdowns of the nutrient value of a wide array of common foods. I think foods will differ depending on where and how they are grown but at least this provides a ballpark guide.

Another tool that will be very useful is diet tracking tool. One that you can enter your daily consumption and get a tally of the nutrient and mineral totals for that day. Again these figures will be a ballpark guide to see if you are on track.

There are loads of online tools for this purpose and one suggestion is https://cronometer.com. I found it easy to use and the tally was fairly comprehensive. Now, it would be a bit of chore to enter everything you eat every day, I suggest using this tool just to find out where you are and what you may be missing or having too much of. Another tool for recipe nutrition data is https://www.verywell.com/recipe-nutrition-analyzer-4129594.

Note that both these tools are USA based so you'll need to find equivalent ingredients in many cases if you are in the UK/AUS.

For recommended daily intakes see https://www.nrv.gov.au / https://ods.od.nih.gov / https://www.nutrition.org.uk

Sodium

Remember most all foods contain sodium, it's not just about how much salt you add. The Australian RDI for sodium is 460-920 mg/day. This figure shouldn't be confused with the recommended upper limit per day which is 2400mg of sodium per day, while the US has an upper limit of 2,300 mg per day and the UK 2400 mg. Confused? So for a healthy person, the recommended daily intake is 460-920 mg/day for good health, and above 2400 mg is likely to cause harm. As discussed earlier, and as your doctor/nutritionist may advise, cutting that sodium intake right back is very advantageous for a person with later stage kidney disease and for blood pressure issues. Such was the case with my father.

When shopping, I read every label and aimed to find foods that contained 120mg per 100g or less of sodium on nutrition labels which I can tell you, is near to impossible for anything processed. Actually, it was a real eye-opener to discover just how much salt is in processed foods.

Phosphorus

Australian RDI 1,000 mg/day and again check the labels and look for 120mg per 100g or less on Nutrition Labels.

Potassium

Australian RDI 3,800 mg/day and again, look for 120mg per 100g or less on Nutrition Labels.

The unfortunate thing is that not many nutrition labels will list phosphorus or potassium, you may have to inquire with the manufacturer or use one of the online tools listed further down in this chapter.

Protein

It's an essential nutrient and the recommended intakes for Men between 19-70 are between 64 and 81g/day, for Women, it's between 46 and 57g/day. Lowering protein intake may be important where the kidney is not functioning correctly and the protein waste is re-entering the bloodstream such as stage 4/5 of CKD. With meat servings, I aimed to keep portion sizes less than palm size as a rough guide.

Here's a brief guide to what we ate more of, and what we ate less of.

Eat More of:

Vegetables

Red Capsicum, Cabbage, Cauliflower, Garlic, Onions. Also OK were Carrots, Celery, Cucumber, Green beans, Lettuce, Watercress, Zucchini, Yellow squash, Asparagus, Radish, Eggplant, Kale, and Turnips.

Fruit

Cranberries, Raspberries, Blueberries, Cherries, Red Grapes and Strawberries. Also OK were Pineapple, Plums, Pears, Apples, Watermelon, and Peaches.

Meat/Bread etc.

Salmon, Red Meat (small serving 1-2 times p/w), Lean Chicken/Pork, Olive oil, Pita bread/Sour-dough/Wholegrain very occasionally, Rice, Sour Cream/Cream Cheese, Greek Yoghurt occasionally.

Eat Less (High Potassium)

Oranges and orange juice, Melons, Apricots, Bananas, Potatoes (cut and boiled OK), Tomatoes, Sweet potatoes, Cooked spinach, Beans (baked, kidney, lima, pinto), Avocado and Kiwi.

Eat Less (High Phosphorus)

Dairy foods (milk, cheese, yogurt) less than 100gm per serve, Beans (baked, kidney, lima, pinto), Nuts and peanut butter, Processed meats (hot dogs, canned meat), Cola, Canned iced teas and lemonade, Bran cereals and Egg yolks.

You can enter and compare foods here http://nutritiondata.self.com by entering favorite fruit or veg, select the portion size which I always choose 100gm to keep to a standard and you can see the full nutrition profile for that item.

Whilst it sounds straightforward enough, it's not easy in real life when you have to make changes. Over the years we all build our own ingrained habits and beliefs, and change is sometimes incredibly difficult. For some people this kind of diet would not to be hard to adjust to, for others it could be mission impossible. It really depends on where you are now as to how difficult it may be to make the changes that may be recommended for you by your nutritionist and doctor.

It's especially hard for carers, who may well know that one type of food is bad, yet if that food is the patients favorite, oh boy, you could be in for a battle! It gets even more difficult with age, a time when we are not so interested in trying new things or making changes as what's delicious is firmly entrenched in our minds.

A few tips on this topic would be to present foods in a recognizable way. If the person's favorite meal outing is a typical meat and veg with sauce all over, then aim to present things in a similar way. Perception is a big part of the game here. If it looks out of the ordinary then it will probably also be rejected as such. Not easy but you'll need to be creative!

Try making adjustments in small steps over a period of

time and you may be lucky in that a complete change may take place without even being noticed.

Another tip is to not try and hold all this in your head, utilize technology or even simple tools to track your progress. A simple way is to track fluids each day by setting up a container and every time you have a drink, add an equal amount of water to the container. At the end of the day, you'll know exactly how much fluid intake you had.

Another tip is to use a photo journal, use your smartphone to take a snap of each meal and at the end of the week, you have a visual diary of your meals to review your progress. No smartphone? A simply written diary does the same thing.

As mentioned earlier, https://cronometer.com is a useful tool for nutrition tracking. Other similar tools include

https://www.supertracker.usda.gov/foodtracker.aspx

http://www.sparkpeople.com/myspark/nutrition_preview.asp

https://www.myfitnesspal.com/

https://www.verywell.com/recipe-nutrition-analyzer-4129594

References:

[1] http://kidney.org.au/your-kidneys/support/kidney-disease/health-and-wellbeing/diet-and-nutrition

[2] http://www.umm.edu/programs/early-renal-insufficiency/health/kidney-disease

[3] http://www.telegraph.co.uk/news/2016/08/31/eating-dinner-after-7pm-may-increase-risk-of-a-heart-attack-stud/

[4] https://www.kidney.org/news/dialysis-health-starts-digestive-tract & https://www.researchgate.net/profile/Fabiola_Martin-Del-Campo

[5] https://www.ncbi.nlm.nih.gov/pubmed/?term=ckd+nutrition

Tips for Daily Life with CKD

Fortunately, there are lots of support programs available. Speak to your doctor about what's available in your local area. Online there are a wealth of resources available via Kidney Health Australia (http://kidney.org.au) or in the US the National Institute for Diabetes and Digestive and Kidney Diseases (https://www.niddk.nih.gov) or in the UK visit Kidney Care UK (https://www.kidneycareuk.org).

Dealing with change, and constantly being in and out of doctors offices and hospitals can be, I should say, IS stressful. Be sure you reach out for support and make yourself available to the support that's on offer even if you think you don't need it. This is not only true for the sufferer but also for carers and family as it will effect everyone's life to some degree.

Be flexible

The trips to doctors, tests, in and out of hospital, can all start to feel it's taking over your life, so the need to be flexible is going to be a big help. And sometimes it may feel like every day is something else or another thing in a never ending story. Be flexible and as they say, learn to roll with it. Change is the new constant. And if it gets overwhelming, reach out for support via those contacts you established from your doctor.

Mood and Health

Keeping good mood is a huge help to restoring health and general well-being. Enjoying the simple things in life is a true blessing and finding activities to keep amused, active and engaged is key.

My father was also suffering from arthritis so mobility was an issue, and he was mostly content to simply spend his time sitting at home. Which, if content, is not such a bad thing, being content is almost the holy grail of happiness in some ways. But too much sitting is most definitely not good for health. Keep it moving, even short walks can have huge benefits for mood - *A leisurely walk can boost mood, psychological well-being* - https://www.medicalnewstoday.com/articles/317451.php

Some of our good mood tricks

Keeping the home fresh with plants - life breeds life as they say

Keeping a garden - full of colorful flowers and green grass it brought joy to the eyes. Gardening itself is also a great way to relieve stress.

Books - the library is a treasure trove of stories and information to get engaged with. Reading is a great way to take your mind of things.

Photos – placing memories of loved ones and special times around the home.

Regular walks - Walking can help relieve stress.

Light exercises of a night.

Tips for Being a Carer

My mother was central in the role of being the main career, and what a fantastic job she did. From morning till night. It can be really tough, draining and requires an unparalleled level of commitment and sacrifice. I think an important part of being a carer is knowing when to hand over to someone else, understanding your own limits and being able to access all the help that's available. Let's call it smart caring. It's not helpful if the carers health or well-being also deteriorates. Some suggestions:

- don't try to hold up the world, learn to let go of things
- spread the load and don't try to do everything
- use all the help that's available
- don't let your own health decay
- remember, that you are in a partnership with your doctor, health professionals and community workers, you're not alone.

You and Your Doctor

It's vital to have a great relationship with your doctor and also to respect his constraints. Doctors in these days have patients whizzing in and out of their offices and breakneck speed and if you've sat in those waiting rooms for hours you can understand why they are often hurried.

It's important that you communicate clearly with your doctor and also that the doctor understands your concerns and needs.

It will help enormously if you have familiarised yourself with some of the jargon that relates to kidney disease and are willing to learn. Your doctor can undoubtedly make suggestions for books and literature.

As I stress in other chapters, it's important to be pro-active and to be an active partner in the solution and be willing to participate in solutions. That may mean diet changes, quitting smoking, drinking or other lifestyle changes.

It's also important to be pushing the doctor for all available options and services that may offer assistance, such as a referral to a dietician. Knowing that you are a willing and active participant in your health outcomes can make a big difference to your doctor's approach and your health outcomes.

Finding Stability with CKD

Where are we now? Post departing hospital we learned a lot about a disease that affects so many people and I think we also learned that you have to be proactive, not reactive.

What does that mean to be proactive?

It means taking responsibility for the condition, learning about what your new situation means, learn what you can be doing to achieve better outcomes. Simply throwing it all in the lap of the doctor with the extent of your effort making your way to see him each week is simply not enough.

That really is my takeaway from all of this.

Our current medical system is a very generalized thing, dealing with thousands and thousands of people flowing in and out of its doors every day and doing the best it can to heal as many as it can.

Inside that system are people who are overloaded with duties, career-focused individuals who are obsessed with KPI's and other stats that are going to advance their place in the hierarchy, doctors that are stretched between hospitals and clinics, poor communication and lack of connection to the best and latest information for achieving the best possible outcomes.

That's a long-winded sentence, let me shorten it. It's up to you.

The time in and out of hospital was life-changing for all of us, not to mention stressful. Post hospital was stressful in new ways, not knowing what direction things were going, not knowing what we should or shouldn't be doing, or could be doing. We were lucky that we had a fantastic nephrologist who always put us at ease, and likewise a fantastic local doctor.

We are also fortunate that we live in a country where we have such a highly developed and subsidized medical system. Some countries don't and some people could only dream about the access to medical care that we have.

Even though, the daily life and the outcomes of our situation and my father's heath was, as it should be, a shared outcome. We had to do our part too. And that is the key to success I firmly believe.

How was our outcome?

My father has been stable now for some time. His test results after a period of dipping to new lows started to edge up and most importantly, stabilize. Our Nephrologist hasn't suggested the need for dialysis at this point and that is very comforting. At this stage of my parent's life if we can avoid the need for dialysis I think it will be worth any effort.

A result of our efforts?

I think a combined result beginning with the efforts of the team of doctors when he first went into emergency care, the attention of doctors and nurses in port emergency care, the rehab, the attention of our nephrologist and doctor, combined with our own efforts. Nothing happens in isolation and remember it's always a team effort.

And my Kidney Stones?

I began with that story and I should complete it, in brief at least. I could not get the kidney stone removed while I was in China and simply lived with it for some time. That wasn't a wise choice as the stone was lodged in my ureter and unbeknownst to me at that time it was causing urine to flow back into the kidney along with the ureter walls binding to the stone which would, in turn, make it harder to remove.

On return to Australia and after several operations over a few months the stone was removed. I will never forget what it feels like to have a stent for an extended period, especially one that was causing me so much pain and to urinate so much blood due to ureter wall scaring. Not to mention the pain of the first encounter with the kidney stone trying to move through the ureter, something they say is equivalent to the pain experienced in natural childbirth. A shout out to all the mothers out there, your amazing! Experiencing a 1cm kidney stone, or any stone for that matter, is not something I plan on doing again anytime soon and I continue to be much more focused on fluid intake, reducing weight, and more attention to nutrition and exercise.

CKD Friendly Recipes

In this section, I will share a collection of recipes that are focused on nutrition with a focus on low sodium and no added salt, low potassium and low phosphorus. I am sure you will find they are delicious and nutritious.

I have included a wide range of sauces you can make at home as most store bought sauces are out of the equation due to staggering levels of sodium.

There are a handful of fresh dessert recipes, some mains, salads, and sides.

There is no way it can be everything for everyone, but I hope at least it is a starting point for getting on track and the beginning of a new food journey that can be not only suitable for your condition but nutritious, delicious and health boosting.

I will share a range of online resources to help you find your favorites and discover new ones.

Recipe Resources

https://www.nwkidney.org/living-with-kidney-disease/recipes/

http://www.kidney.org.uk/help-and-info/books/books-foodwiththought/

https://www.davita.com/recipes/

https://www.kidney.org/sites/default/files/docs/kidney_cookbook_lr.pdf [PDF]

http://www.myspiceitup.ca

https://www.kidneyresearchuk.org/file/Cookbook.pdf [PDF]

This is not intended to be your meal plan or a total solution, as everyone has different needs and different tastes. As stated earlier it's key to work with your doctor and dietician to create a plan based on your needs and, importantly, foods and dishes that you are also going to enjoy.

The intention here with these recipes is to inspire and to say, hey, this is doable!

Conventions used are

tsp = teaspoon

tsbp = tablespoon

g = gram

oz = ounce

fl oz = us fluid ounce

Skillet = frying pan.

250 ml = 1 cup

175 ml = 3/4 cup

125 ml = 1/2 cup

60 ml = 1/4 cup

15 ml = 1 tablespoon (Tbsp)

5 ml = 1 teaspoon (tsp)

Mains

Salmon with Mustard-Wine Sauce

Ingredients:

1 tsp minced garlic

1/2 tsp salt

1 tsp freshly ground black pepper, divided

2 tbsps. olive oil

2 tbsps. fresh lemon juice

2 tbsps. butter

1 tbsp. flour

1/2 tsp paprika

3/4 cup milk

2 tbsps. Dijon mustard1/4 cup dry white wine

1 tsp chopped fresh basil leaves

1 tsp chopped fresh rosemary leaves

Method:

In a small bowl, combine garlic, salt, 1/2 tsp. pepper, the oil, and lemon juice.

Brush mixture over salmon, then cook, turning once, until done the way you like, about 6 minutes total for medium.

In a small saucepan, melt butter over medium heat.

Stir in flour and cook until starting to brown.

Whisk in remaining 1/2 tsp. pepper, the paprika, milk, mustard, wine, and 3 tbsp. water.

Cook until simmering. Spoon over salmon and sprinkle with herbs.

Rosemary Chicken Thighs with Garlic Kale

Ingredients:

1 garlic clove, pressed

1 tbsp. olive oil

2 tbsps. Dijon mustard

2 tbsps. honey

1 tsp chopped fresh rosemary

1/2 tsp pepper

450 g/1.5 pounds skinless, boneless chicken thighs

1/2 lemon

Sautéed Garlic Kale (see Sides Recipes)

Method:

Combine garlic, oil, mustard, honey, rosemary and pepper in a large heavy-duty zip-top plastic bag, squeezing bag to combine ingredients. Add chicken, turning to coat, and seal bag. Chill for 1 to 24 hours.

Preheat grill to 175 C/350 F (medium-high). Remove chicken from marinade, discarding marinade.

Grill chicken, covered with grill lid, for 5 to 7 minutes on each side. Transfer chicken to a large piece of aluminium foil. Squeeze juice from lemon over chicken; fold foil around chicken, covering chicken completely. Allow to stand for 10 minutes while you prepare the Sautéed Garlic Kale (see Sides Recipes).

Serve together and enjoy.

Coconut Mango Chicken

Ingredients:

1 egg

1/2 cup shredded unsweetened coconut

4-6 ounces (113 g) skinless, boneless chicken breasts

3 tbsps. vegetable oil

Method:

Preheat the oven to 350 (175C) degrees.

Prepare the Mango Salsa as per the recipe in the Meat Sauces, Dipping Sauces and Gravies section.

Beat the egg with 1 tsp water. Dip the chicken in the egg mix, then in the coconut lightly pressing to ensure a good coat.

In large skillet (pan) heat the oil over medium-high heat. Add the chicken, turning once, cooking until golden or about 3 minutes. Transfer to an oven pan and bake until cooked through, about 12 minutes.

Serve the chicken with the mango salsa and a few green salad leaves as desired.

Baked Yoghurt Chicken with Tomato, Mint and Cucumber Salad

Ingredients:

1/2 tsp Chinese five-spice powder

1 tsp chilli powder

2 tsps. soy sauce

1 clove garlic, crushed

1 tbsp. olive oil

200 g reduced-fat natural yoghurt

4 x 200 g skinless chicken breasts

Salad:

2 Lebanese (small) cucumbers, sliced

4 Roma (plum) tomatoes, sliced

1/2 red (Spanish) onion, finely sliced

1/4 cup mint leaves

1 tbsp. olive oil

1 tsp lemon juice

Method:

In a bowl, gently fold five-spice powder, chilli powder, soy sauce, garlic and oil through yoghurt. Coat chicken with mixture and allow to stand at least 4 hours.

Preheat oven to 180C (356F). Line a baking dish with baking

paper.

Heat a non-stick frying pan over medium heat. Add chicken and cook for 2 minutes each side. Transfer to prepared baking dish and bake for 6-8 minutes, or until cooked through. Remove and allow chicken to rest for 5 minutes. Carve into thick slices.

To make the salad gently toss all ingredients. Divide between four serving plates, then add chicken and serve.

Crumbed Salmon with Asparagus and Baby Red Potatoes

Ingredients:

1/2 cup breadcrumbs

1/3 cup basil leaves

3 tbsps. grated parmesan cheese

1 1/2 tbsps. olive oil

3 salmon fillets, skin on

6 asparagus

6 baby red potatoes, quartered

Method:

Preheat oven to 200c/190 (400F) fan forced

Combine breadcrumbs, basil, parmesan and olive oil, and blitz in a blender

Add a little olive oil to a roasting pan and add fillets, add the crumb mixture to the top of the fillets

Place into hot oven for 10-15 minutes.

In the meantime, place the potatoes into a saucepan with 2L (67 fl oz) water, a garlic clove and rosemary sprig, and bring to the boil. When the potatoes are nearly done, at about 6 minutes, cut the woody end of the asparagus, and blanch for 2-3 minutes.

Remove the salmon from the oven and add to the plate, add asparagus to the plate, add potatoes to the plate, add a little butter atop the potatoes and sprinkle with rosemary. Serve with a little tartare sauce.

Poached Salmon with Lemon Parsley Sauce

Ingredients:

1 large white onion, thickly sliced

2 dried bay leaves

4 whole black peppercorns

1 cup dry white wine

4 (180g/6.4 oz) salmon fillets, skin removed

20g/.7 oz butter

1 tbsp. plain flour

1 cup (240 ml/8.1 fl oz) low-fat milk

1/4 cup finely-chopped flat-leaf parsley leaves

1 1/2 tbsps. lemon juice

Method:

Combine onion, bay leaves, peppercorns, wine and 3 cups of cold water in a large, deep frying pan or saucepan. Bring to a simmer over medium heat.

Add fish (adding more water to cover fish, if required). Simmer, uncovered, for 5 minutes or until fish is just cooked through. Remove from heat. Cover pan. Set aside.

Meanwhile, melt butter in a saucepan over medium-low heat. Add flour. Cook, stirring, for 1 minute. Gradually stir in milk. Increase heat to medium. Cook, stirring, for 3 minutes or until sauce thickens and coats the back of a wooden spoon. Remove from heat. Stir in parsley and lemon juice.

Using a slotted spoon, remove fish to plates. Drizzle with lemon parsley sauce. Season with pepper.

Serve with broccolini.

Country Gravy

Ingredients:

8 ounces ground pork, uncooked

3/4 tsp ground sage

1/2 tsp round basil

1/2 tsp black pepper

1/4 tsp fennel seeds

1/8 tsp crushed red pepper flakes

2 tbsps. cornstarch

1-1/3 cups liquid nondairy creamer

2 tbsps. unsalted margarine

Method:

In a medium bowl, mix ground pork with sage, basil, pepper, fennel seeds and pepper.

Brown the pork mixture in a skillet over medium heat. Drain, remove from pan and set aside.

In a small bowl, mix cornstarch with 1/3-cup creamer and stir until smooth.

Melt margarine over low heat in the same skillet used for cooking the pork. Add cornstarch mixture and remaining nondairy creamer to margarine and cook over low heat, stirring constantly, until mixture thickens and bubbles.

Add pork and heat thoroughly. Serve over a hot biscuit or toasted bread.

Orange-Glazed Chicken

Ingredients:

1/4 cup (60 ml/2 fl oz) olive oil

6 Chicken Breast Halves

2 tbsps. Flour

1/8 tsp Nutmeg

1 dash Ginger

1/4 tsp Cinnamon

1 1/2 cup (350 ml/11.8 fl oz) Orange Juice

1/4 cup Raisins

1/2 cup Mandarin Orange (Optional)

Method:

Heat oil in a non-stick large fry pan. Brown chicken on both side. Remove chicken and set aside.

Blend flour, nutmeg, ginger, and cinnamon together; add mixture to hot oil. Whisk together quickly to make a smooth paste.

Gradually add orange juice to pan. Stir constantly.

Cook over medium heat until soft thicken for 3 mins. Return chicken to pan.

Add raisin, cook in low heat for 30 mins or till chicken tender or fully cooked. Add water to soft if thickens too much.

Add mandarin orange slice and heat until warm.

Serve with your favourite salad, or rice and/or steamed greens.

Spicy Chicken Breasts with Cabbage

Ingredients:

4 Chicken breasts

1 tsp ground coriander

1 tsp ground turmeric

1/2 tsp paprika

2 tsps. cumin seeds

3 Spring onions. chopped

1 small wombok cabbage

2 tbsps. chopped cilantro leaves

Squeeze of lemon juice

Method:

Preheat oven to 180 C/355 F (160 C/320 F for fan forced ovens).

Mix coriander, paprika, pepper and turmeric, rub spice mixture all over the chicken

In a hot pan, sear the chicken breasts for about 3 minutes a side, until golden brown, about 6 minutes total, and set aside.

Add the spring onions to the pan, sprinkle over the cumin, cook on a medium heat until softened, about 1 minute. Add the cabbage and combine, heat for another 2 minutes.

Place the cabbage mix into a baking pan and place the chicken fillets amongst it and place in the oven for about 15 minutes.

Sprinkle with the chopped cilantro, lemon juice, and pepper.

Italian Meatballs

Ingredients:

1.3 kg/3 pounds ground beef

3 large eggs, beaten

1 cup dry oatmeal flakes

6 tbsps. parmesan cheese

1 tbsp. olive oil

1 tbsp. garlic powder

2 tsps. dried oregano

1 cup onion, chopped

1 tsp. black pepper

Method:

Preheat oven to 375 degrees.

Combine all ingredients in a large bowl and mix together.

Roll into 1″ balls and place on a baking sheet.

Bake for 10 to 15 minutes, until meatballs are cooked through.

To serve, place meatballs in a warming dish or crock pot on low heat setting. Serve with 2 teaspoons sauce on the side.

Serve together with a Greek Salad or Caesar Salad.

Broccoli Chicken Casserole

Ingredients:

2-3 cups cooked broccoli

1 medium onion, chopped

2-3 chicken breast, diced

2 tbsps. butter or margarine

2 eggs, beaten

2 cups milk

2 cups cooked rice, barley, or noodles

2 cups grated cheese

to top grated parmesan

Method:

Cook broccoli in microwave.

Meanwhile, brown onion and chicken in butter in a pan.

Mix all ingredients and put in greased casserole dish.

Sprinkle top with grated parmesan and bake about 1 hour and 15 minutes at 350 degrees, until set and fork comes out clean.

Roast Chicken with Cumin Honey and Orange

Ingredients:

1/2 cup (120 ml/4 fl oz) freshly squeezed orange juice

1/2 cup (120 ml4 fl oz) honey

1 tbsp. ground cumin

Salt and freshly ground black pepper

1 3-pound chicken, giblets and excess fat removed

Method:

Preheat oven to 400 (200 C) degrees. Use a non-stick roasting pan, or line a roasting pan with a double layer of aluminium foil. Combine orange juice, honey, cumin, salt and pepper in bowl, and whisk until smooth. Place chicken in pan, and spoon all but 1/4 cup of liquid over all of it.

Place chicken in oven, legs first, and roast for 10 minutes. Spoon accumulated juices back over chicken, reverse pan back to front, and return to oven. Repeat four times, basting every 10 minutes and switching pan position each time. If chicken browns too quickly, lower heat a bit. If juices dry up, use reserved liquid and 1 or 2 tablespoons of water or orange juice.

After 50 minutes of roasting, insert an instant-read thermometer into a thigh; when it reads 155 to 165 degrees, remove chicken from oven, and baste one final time. Let rest 5 minutes before serving.

Serve with your choice of veg such as Healthy Herbed Veg or Sauteed Garlic Kale.

Smoked Salmon and Asparagus Frittata

Ingredients:

12 spears asparagus (preferably thin stemmed), trimmed

8 eggs

3 tbsps. chopped dill

200 g smoked salmon, cut into strips

50 g grated parmesan

Method:

Preheat the oven to 150 C/302 F. Line a 20-cm square cake tin with baking paper.

Bring a large saucepan of water to the boil, add the asparagus and cook until just tender. Drain and rinse under cold water, then cut into 1 cm length.

Whisk together the eggs and dill in the bowl. Season, then stir in the asparagus and smoked salmon. Pour into the prepared tin and sprinkle with grated parmesan. Bake for 25 minutes or until just set. Remove from the oven and allow to cool.

Cut into pieces and serve with Asparagus Salad.

Corn Fritters with Smoked Salmon and Spinach

Ingredients:

1 cup (160 g/5.6 fl oz) wholemeal self-raising flour

2 eggs

1 cup (250 ml/8.4 fl oz) buttermilk

125 g/4.4 oz of cooked corn kernals

4 spring onions (scallions), finely sliced

1/4 cup roughly chopped flat-leaf (Italian) parsley

1/2 red capsicum (pepper), seeded and finely diced

1 tbsp. lemon juice

1/2 cup (140 g/4.9 oz) reduced-fat natural yoghurt

1/4 cup roughly chopped coriander (cilantro) leaves

1 tbsp. olive oil

300 g/10.5 oz smoked salmon

100 g/3.5 oz baby spinach

Method:

In a large bowl, sift flour and make a well in the centre. In a separate bowl, mix eggs and buttermilk. Pour egg mixture into flour and stir to make a smooth batter. Add corn, spring onions, parsley and capsicum and fold through.

In a small bowl, mix lemon juice, yoghurt and coriander, and set aside.

Heat oil in a large non-stick frying pan over medium heat. Drop 1/3-cupfuls of mixture into the pan and cook for 3 minutes, or until golden. Turn and cook for a further 3 minutes, or until mixture is firm and set.

Serve fritters with the smoked salmon and spinach, drizzled with a little yogurt dressing.

Char-Grilled Salmon with Asparagus and Pumpkin

Ingredients:

400 g/14 oz butternut pumpkin, peeled and thickly sliced

1 tbsp. olive oil

4 x 200 g/7 oz salmon fillets

16 spears asparagus

1/3 cup (110 g/3.9 oz) Parsley Relish

lime wedges

Method:

Preheat oven to 180C (356F).

See Meat Sauces, Dipping Sauces and Gravies for Parsley Relish recipe.

Place pumpkin in a bowl with half the oil and toss to coat. Transfer to a baking dish and lightly season. Bake for 20 minutes, or until soft and golden.

Meanwhile, heat a non-stick grill plate or barbecue grill to high.

Lightly brush salmon fillets with remaining oil. Place salmon on grill, flesh-side down, and cook for 4 minutes. Turn salmon and cook for a further 4 minutes. Remove from heat and set aside, covered.

Bring a saucepan of water to a boil. Add asparagus and blanch for 2 minutes, then drain. Arrange salmon on pumpkin slices, then top with parsley relish and add asparagus spears. Serve with lime wedges.

Chicken and Tarragon meatloaf

Ingredients:

1 1/2 tbsps. olive oil

1 small Granny Smith apple, peeled and diced

1 onion, finely chopped

1 clove garlic, finely chopped

1 tbsp. tarragon, finely chopped

2 slices bread, crumbled into breadcrumbs

1 egg, lightly beaten

3 spring onions (scallions), finely sliced

1 small zucchini (courgette), grated

1 tbsp. fruit chutney

1 kg lean minced (ground) chicken

Method:

Preheat oven to 150C (302F). Lightly grease a loaf tin.

Heat oil in a large frying pan over medium heat. Add apple, onion and garlic and cook for 8 minutes, or until soft and golden.

In a large bowl, combine onion mixture, tarragon, breadcrumbs, egg, spring onion, zucchini, chutney and chicken. Lightly season. Spoon into prepared loaf tin and bake for 1 hour. Allow to cool in the tin, then turn out onto your work surface and cut into 5 thick slices.

Serve with salad.

Chargrilled Pesto Chicken with Tabouleh

Ingredients:

4 x 200 g/7 oz skinless chicken breast fillets

1 lemon, cut into wedges

Pesto

1 cup loosely packed basil leaves

1 clove garlic, crushed

1 tbsp. lemon juice

1 tbsp. olive oil

1 tbsp. pine nuts

tabouleh (see Salads section)

Method:

Place pesto ingredients in a food processor and blend to a coarse paste.

Rub pesto into chicken. Preheat a grill plate or barbecue grill to high. Cook chicken for 6 minutes each side, or until cooked through.

Slice chicken and serve with tabouleh and lemon wedges and a side salad.

Stuffed Baked Chicken Breast

Ingredients:

2 spring onions (scallions), finely sliced

150 g/5.2 oz reduced-fat ricotta

finely grated zest of 1 lemon

1/4 cup chopped flat-leaf (Italian) parsley

1 tbsp. lemon juice

1/4 cup pine nuts, lightly toasted

4 x 180 g/6.3 oz skinless chicken breast fillets

1 tbsp. olive oil

Method:

In a small bowl, combine the spring onions, ricotta, lemon zest and juice, parsley and pine nuts. Season lightly, then cover and refrigerate for 10 minutes.

Meanwhile, with a sharp knife, make a long incision along the side and into the centre of each chicken breast, being careful not to cut through to the other side.

Spoon a quarter of the ricotta mixture into each breast.

Preheat oven to 180C (356F).

Heat oil in a frying pan over high heat. Add chicken and cook for 4 minutes each side, then transfer to a baking tray. Bake for 10 minutes, or until cooked through.

Serve chicken with mixed steamed vegetables such as Healthy Herbed Mix Veg.

Pork with Roasted Pears and Creamed Greens

Ingredients:

olive oil spray

4 small pears, halved and cored

1 tbsp. balsamic vinegar

800 g/28 oz pork fillets, trimmed of fat

Creamed greens:

200 g/7 oz baby spinach leaves

1 bunch watercress, washed and trimmed, leaves coarsely chopped

large handful rocket, coarsely chopped

2/3 cup (160 ml/5.4 fl oz) reduced-fat evaporated milk

3 tsps. cornflour (corn-starch)

Method:

Preheat the oven to 180C (356F).

Spray the base of a small roasting tin with olive oil. Add the pears, cut-side down, then roast for 35 minutes or until tender.

Meanwhile, spray a large ovenproof frying pan with olive oil, then heat over medium-high heat. Add the pork fillets and cook, turning often, for 3-4 minutes or until browned all over. Transfer the pan to the oven, then roast for 15 minutes or until cooked through but still a little pink in the middle.

To make the creamed greens, place the spinach, watercress and rocket in a large saucepan with 2 tbsps. water. Cover the pan, then cook over medium-high heat for 4-5 minutes or until the spinach has wilted. Add the milk and bring to the boil. Combine the cornflour with 1 tbsp water in a small bowl to form a smooth paste. Stirring constantly, add the paste to the pan and cook until the liquid boils and thickens. Season to taste with salt and pepper.

Cut the pork into thick slices, then serve with the roasted pears and creamed greens.

Rosemary Roast Chicken and Veg

Ingredients:

2 medium zucchini

1 medium carrots

1/2 red capsicum

1/2 large red onion

8 garlic cloves

1 tbsp. olive oil

1/4 tsp ground pepper

4 chicken breasts

1 tbsp. dried rosemary

Method:

Preheat the oven to 200 C/390 F or 180 C/356 F fan forced.

Slice the zucchini 1cm thick; slice the carrot 1/2cm thick; cut onion and capsicum into wedges; crush garlic cloves.

Combine the zucchini, carrot, capsicum, onion, garlic and oil in a roasting pan. Season the mixture with 1/2 tsp black pepper and toss to coat.

Mix pepper and rosemary together with a little olive oil and rub over chicken.

Place onto pan with veggies, and into the oven for about 35 minutes or until the chicken is cooked through.

Chicken with Cranberry braised red cabbage

Ingredients:

1 tbsp. olive oil

1 red cabbage, finely shredded

120 g (4 oz) dried cranberries

1 1/2 cups (375 ml/12.6 fl oz) cranberry juice

1 sprig rosemary

4 x 200 g (7 oz) skinless chicken breast fillets

1 quantity Cauliflower Carrot Mash

Method:

Heat some oil in a large saucepan (skillet) over low-medium heat.

Add the cabbage, then cover and cook, stirring often, for 10 minutes or until wilted. Add the cranberries, cranberry juice and rosemary and cook, stirring often, for 20 minutes or until the cabbage is tender and the liquid has reduced. Discard the rosemary.

Meanwhile, preheat the oven to 200 C (392 F). Spray a baking dish with olive oil, place the chicken in and cover the dish tightly with foil. Bake for 8 minutes, then remove from the oven and leave to stand, covered, for 5 minutes; the chicken should be cooked through.

Season to taste and cut into thick slices. Divide the cabbage, chicken and mash among plates and serve.

Honey-Mustard Pork with Warm Cabbage Salad

Ingredients:

800 g/28 oz pork fillet, trimmed of fat and cut into 4 cm slices

olive oil spray

1/4 cup (60 ml/2 fl oz) chicken stock/chicken broth

1/4 cup (90 g/3.17 oz) honey mustard

1/4 cup (60 g/2.11 oz) sour cream

Warm cabbage salad:

1 tbsp. olive oil

2 cups (160 g/5.6 oz) shredded red cabbage

2 carrots, grated

3 spring onions, sliced

1 1/2 cup (125 ml/4.2 fl oz) white wine vinegar

Method:

Heat a a pan over medium heat and cook the pork for 3-4 minutes each side and remove from the pan, cover with foil and keep warm.

Add the stock to the pan and stir. Then add the mustard and sour cream and continue stirring until combined and heated through.

In another pan, heat the olive oil and add the cabbage, carrot and spring onion. Cook until softened and stir in the vinegar.

Add the pork to the serving plate and drizzle with the prepared sauce alongside a portion of the cabbage salad.

Greek Lamb Kebabs with tzatziki

Ingredients:

800 g/28.2 oz lamb fillets, cut into cubes

1 red capsicum/bell pepper, cut into squares

1 Green capsicum/bell pepper, cut into squares

1 red Spanish onion, cut into squares

Marinade:

2 tbsps. dried oregano

1 tbsp. olive oil

1 clove garlic, crushed

Tzatziki:

1 clove garlic, crushed

200 g/7 oz greek yoghurt

1 Lebanese (small) or continental cucumber, finely grated

1/2 red (Spanish) onion, finely diced

1 tbsp. chopped flat-leaf (Italian) parsley

1 tbsp. chopped mint

Method:

Mix the olive oil, oregano and garlic in a bowl and add lamb, turning to coat. Cover with plastic wrap and refrigerate for 2 hours or overnight.

Preheat grill plate or barbecue grill to high.

Thread lamb, peppers/capsicum and onion onto skewers. Grill for 2 minutes each side for a total of about 8 minutes.

Meanwhile, combine all tzatziki ingredients in a bowl and lightly season. Serve alongside kebabs along with a Greek Salad or Cucumber Salad.

Creamy Cauliflower and Coconut Curry

Ingredients:
2 tbsps. coconut oil

1 large head of cauliflower (about 800 g/28 oz), cut into bite-sized florets

1 onion, chopped

1 tsp finely grated ginger

2 garlic cloves, chopped

1 tsp mustard seeds

11/2 tbsps. garam masala

11/2 tsps. ground turmeric

1-2 pinches of cayenne pepper (optional)

15 fresh curry leaves

600 ml/20 fl oz coconut cream

200 ml/6.7 fl oz water

black pepper

juice of 1 lemon

Method:
Heat 1 tbsp. of the oil or fat in a large frying pan over medium-high heat. Add the cauliflower in batches and cook for 5 minutes until lightly golden. Remove the cauliflower from the pan.

Add the remaining oil and the onion to the pan and cook, stirring occasionally, for 5 minutes, or until the onion is translucent. Add the ginger, garlic and mustard seeds and cook, stirring constantly, for 20-30 seconds until the mustard seeds start to pop. Reduce the heat to medium-low, stir in the ground spices and cook for 15 seconds until fragrant.

Add the curry leaves to the pan and cook for 10 seconds. Pour in the coconut cream and water, return the cauliflower to the pan and stir to combine.

Reduce the heat to low, cover with a lid and cook for 30 minutes until the cauliflower is tender and the sauce has thickened slightly.

Season with pepper. Stir through the lemon juice and serve.

Zucchini Frittata

Ingredients:

2 tbsps. olive oil

1 shallot, finely chopped

1 medium zucchini, diced

6 eggs

2 tbsps. milk, or water

1/4 cup freshly grated Parmigiano-Reggiano

Freshly ground black pepper

1 tbsp. unsalted butter

2 to 3 zucchini flowers, cleaned, stamen removed and torn in half, optional

Method:

Heat the oil in a small pan over medium heat and add the shallots and zucchini. Cook until just beginning to soften, about 3 to 4 minutes.

Beat the eggs with the milk and add the parmigiano and a sprinkle of pepper. Stir until combined.

Add the zucchini to the eggs and stir to combine.

Add the butter to saucepan, melt, and add the egg and zucchini mixture. Cover the pan and cook over medium-low heat until the edges of the frittata begin to brown and the centre has set, about 8 minutes.

Turn out onto a cutting board slice into pieces and serve alongside your favorite salad.

Sides

Cauliflower Faux Potato Mash

Ingredients

1 head of cauliflower

3 tablespoons milk

1 tablespoon butter

2 tablespoons light sour cream

1/4 teaspoon garlic powder

freshly ground black pepper

snipped chives

Method:

Separate the cauliflower into florets and chop the core finely.

Bring about 1 cup of water to a simmer in a pot, then add the cauliflower. Cover and turn the heat to medium. Cook the cauliflower for 12-15 minutes or until very tender.

Drain and discard all of the water and add the milk, butter, sour cream, garlic powder, pepper and mash.

Top with the chives.

Cauliflower Carrot Mash

Ingredients:

1 head of cauliflower

3 medium carrots

1 sweet onion, chopped

2 cloves garlic, minced

1 tablespoon fresh rosemary, minced

1 tablespoon fresh thyme, minced

2 tablespoons olive oil

pepper to taste

Method:

Chop the cauliflower into florets, chop the carrots into bite size pieces, along with the garlic and onion.

Place cauliflower and carrots in a steamer basket, season with pepper, and steam until soft, about 10 minutes.

Heat 1 tablespoon olive oil in non-stick skillet (frying pan) on medium heat.

Saute onion, garlic, and herbs until onion is translucent. Don't burn the garlic! Set aside.

Place steamed cauliflower and carrots into a food processor along with the onion, garlic, herbs, plus the olive oil. Process until you have a desired smooth consistency.

Garnish as you please and serve.

Quick Pressure Cooker Coconut Rice

Ingredients:

1 1/2 cups Jasmine Rice

1 can (14 ounces/400 g) Coconut Milk

1/2 cup water

1 tsp sugar

Method:

Rinse rice in cool water until the water runs clear. Drain the rice in a colander or sieve.

Add the rice, coconut milk, water, sugar and salt to the pressure cooker pot. Stir. Lock lid in place.

Select high pressure and 3 minutes cook time. When timer beeps, turn pressure cooker off and let the pressure release naturally.

After 7 minutes release any remaining pressure.

Fluff rice with a fork. Spoon rice into serving bowl.

Red Cabbage with Apples

Ingredients:

1 Onion (coarsely chopped)

2 tbsps. Olive oil

1/4 cup Cider vinegar

2 tbsps. Brown sugar

1 Green apple (cored and thinly sliced)

1 small head Red cabbage (coarsely shredded)

pepper to taste

Method:

In a large skillet, sauté onion in oil until softened (approximately 5 minutes).

Mix in vinegar, sugar, and pepper. Add cabbage and apple.

Bring to a boil, reduce heat, cover, and simmer until cabbage wilts (approximately 10 minutes), stirring occasionally.

Dilled Carrots

Ingredients:

450 g/1 lb Carrots

1 1/2 cups White vinegar

1/2 cup Plain rice vinegar

2 tsps. Dill weed

3 tbsps. Sugar

1/4 tsps. Pepper

2 tsps. Garlic powder or fresh garlic

Method:

Cut the carrots into small strips.

Steam in the microwave about 3 to 5 minutes.

Cool the carrots by plunging them into ice water.

Mix all the ingredients.

Pour over carrots.

Place in a covered container and chill overnight.

Red Cabbage with Cranberries

Ingredients:

3 tbsps. olive oil

2 large onion, halved and thinly sliced

1 tsp ground cloves

1 medium red cabbage, quartered, cored and thinly sliced

200ml vegetable stock

3 tbsps. balsamic vinegar

100g brown sugar

200g fresh or frozen cranberry

Method:

Heat the oil in a large pan. Add the onions and fry, stirring every now and then, for about 10 mins, until they start to caramelise.

Stir in the cloves, then add the cabbage and continue cooking, stirring more frequently this time, until the cabbage starts to soften.

Pour in the stock, add the vinegar and sugar, then cover and cook for 10 mins.

Stir in the cranberries and cook for 10 mins more. Cool and keep in the fridge for up to 4 days, or freeze for 1 month. Thaw in the fridge overnight. Reheat until very hot before serving

Sautéed Red Cabbage

Ingredients:

2 tbsps. olive oil

1 small onion, sliced

1/2 red cabbage, shredded

1/3 cup white vinegar

2 tbsps sugar

1 tsp mustard seed

pepper

Method:

Heat a skillet (frying pan) over medium high heat.

Add oil and onion and sauté 2 minutes.

Add cabbage and turn in pan, sautéing it until it wilts, 3 to 5 minutes.

Add vinegar to the pan and turn the cabbage in it.

Sprinkle sugar over the cabbage and turn again.

Season with mustard seed and pepper and reduce the heat to low.

Continue to cook 8 minutes, stirring occasionally.

Healthy Herbed Mix Veg

Ingredients:

3 Red Potato, quartered

1/2 Cauliflower Head, sectioned into small florets

3 Summer Squash, sliced

1 Zucchini, sliced

1/2 Broccoli Head (or one small head), sectioned into bite size florets

3 tbsps. butter

1 tbsp. olive oil

2 tsp The Dish Seasoning

Method:

Place potatoes into pot and fill with cold water, add thyme, garlic and bring to a boil.

Once boiling, add other vegetables and lower heat to a simmer for 5-7 minutes.

Remove from heat and strain and cover to keep warm.

Drain pot and remove vegetables. Add butter, olive oil and dish seasoning to pot, allow to melt and pour over plated vegetables.

Simple Boiled Butter Potatoes

Ingredients:

450 g/1 lb small new potatoes

1 head garlic, halved crosswise

1 bay leaf

1 tsp black peppercorns

2 to 4 tbsps. unsalted butter

Freshly ground black pepper

Method:

Put the potatoes, garlic, bay leaf, and peppercorns in a large saucepan, add cold water to cover by about an inch.

Bring to a boil, lower the heat, and simmer until potatoes are fork tender, about 5 to 8 minutes depending on their size.

Drain and discard the garlic, bay leaves, and peppercorns.

Halve the potatoes, if large, toss with the butter and season with and pepper, to taste. Keep warm.

Spicy Roasted Cauliflower

Ingredients:

1 small or half large cauliflower, cut into florets

1 tbsp. olive oil

1 tbsp. Baharat spice mix (see Sauces, Spices and Rubs)

Yoghurt sauce , to serve (see Sauces, Spices and Rubs)

Method:

Preheat the oven to 200C (392F) and line a baking tray with baking paper.

Combine the cauliflower, olive oil and spice mix in a bowl and toss to coat. Place the cauliflower on the tray in a single layer and roast for 30 minutes or until well coloured, turning once or twice.

Serve with a dollop of Yoghurt sauce (optional)

Roasted and Marinated Capsicum

Ingredients:
1 Capsicum (pepper), red or green
1 tbsp. Olive oil
Rosemary Sprig
1 clove Garlic, sliced
2 tbsps. Olive oil

Method:
Preheat the oven to 200c (392F).

Wash the whole capsicum and dry well. Place the capsicum on a flat oven tray.

Pour the 1 tbsp oil over the top and place in the preheated oven for approximately 20 minutes, turning occasionally to get even colouring.

Remove the capsicum from the oven, place it in a bowl and cover with plastic film wrap for 20 minutes.

Mix the olive oil, garlic and rosemary together in a small bowl.

Peel the skin off the outside of the capsicum, split open lengthwise and remove the seeds and ribs.

Cut the capsicum into long wide strips and immerse in the olive oil marinade until needed.

Sautéed Jerusalem Artichoke

Ingredients:
220 g/7.7 oz Jerusalem artichokes
1 tsp White vinegar
2 cups Water
2 Scallions (spring onions), chopped
1 tbsp. Ginger, fresh grated
1 tbsp. butter

Method:

Place the artichokes in a pan and barely cover with the water and vinegar.

Bring the pot to the boil and continue to simmer until the artichokes become tender.

Drain the liquid away and allow to cool and then rub the skins off under cold running water.

Slice the artichokes into even discs.

Add the butter to a fry pan and heat on the stove. Add the sliced artichokes and ginger and sauté until they change colour slightly.

Add the chopped spring onions and seasoning, toss in the pan and serve.

Simple Boiled Eggs

Ingredients:
3 cups Water
2 tbsps. White vinegar
5 Eggs

Method:
In a large pot bring the water and vinegar to the boil.

Lower the eggs into the boiling water and cook as desired:
soft boiled 3-4 minutes
medium boiled 5-6 minutes
hard boiled 9-10 minutes.

Noting that the cooking time starts when the water returns to the boil.

If not eating immediately, refrigerate eggs until they are completely cold and use in salads etc.

Poached eggs

Ingredients:
Water 1.5 L
White vinegar 15 ml (1 tbsp)
Eggs 5

Method:
Bring the water and vinegar to the boil.

Break the eggs into individual bowls to check for blood or broken yolks.

Gently slide one egg at a time into the simmering poaching liquid. Allow 15-20 seconds between each egg for the water to regain temperature.

Adjust the temperature to just below simmering and poach for 3 minutes or until the white is firm and the yolks are still runny, yet warm.

Remove the eggs and serve hot.

Simple Braised Veg

Ingredients:
2 tbsps. olive oil

1 onion, cut into 1 cm thick wedges

3 garlic cloves, finely sliced

10 Dutch carrots, leafy tips trimmed

6 radishes, halved

3 turnips, cut into 3 cm pieces

1/4 savoy cabbage, roughly chopped

1 green apple, cored and cut into 2.5cm pieces

l cup Chicken Bone Broth or water

2 bay leaves

freshly ground black pepper

Method:
Preheat the oven to 180C (356F).

Add the oil to a large flameproof casserole dish over medium heat. Add the onion and garlic and cook for 2 minutes until starting to colour slightly.

Add the carrots, radish, turnip, cabbage and apple and cook, stirring occasionally, for 6 minutes until just starting to colour.

Pour in the broth or water, add the bay leaves and season with pepper. Cover with a lid or some foil and braise in the oven for 30 minutes until the vegetables are tender.

Transfer to a serving dish.

Zucchini rice

Ingredients:
2 large zucchini
1 tsp coconut oil

Method:
Slice off the ends of the zucchini and discard.

Slice them into long, thin strips and then cut into tiny pieces the size of rice grains.

Heat the oil in a wok or frying pan over medium heat. Add the zucchini rice and sauté for 5 minutes until softened.

Buttered carrots

Ingredients:
300 g/10.5 oz Carrots
1 tbps. Butter, melted
t tsp Parsley, chopped

Method:
Peel the carrots and wash them.

Cut into even sized pieces about 4 cm long.

Place in cold water and bring to boil with the lid on. Cook for 20 minutes or until just tender.

Drain well and toss in melted butter.

Dress into hot serving dishes and sprinkle with chopped parsley.

Sautéed Garlic Kale

450 g/1.5 lb young kale, stems and leaves coarsely chopped

3 tbsps olive oil

2 cloves garlic, finely sliced

1/2 cup vegetable stock or water

pepper

2 tbsps red wine vinegar

Heat olive oil in a large saucepan over a low heat. Add the garlic and cook gently until soft, being careful not to burn or discolor.

Add the stock and kale and toss to combine and raise the heat. Cover and cook for 5 minutes.

Remove cover and continue to cook, stirring until all the liquid has evaporated. Add the vinegar and season with pepper to taste.

Soups

Simple Chinese Pork and Corn Soup

Ingredients:

700 g/24.6 oz pork bones or pork ribs

1 sweet corn, cut into thirds

1 large carrot, peeled and cut into 2 cm pieces

2 medium turnips or radish, peeled and cut into 2 cm pieces

Method:

Blanch pork bones by bringing a pot of water to the boil, drop the bones in for about a few minutes. Drain and rinse pork under cold water.

Bring 2 L/67 fl oz water to the boil and add all ingredients. Once it's returned to the boil then reduce to a low simmer. Leave it to simmer for around an hour, a little earlier or later is OK too.

Chicken and Vegetable Comfort Soup

Ingredients:

2 tbsps. olive oil

1 onion chopped

3 garlic cloves, finely chopped

1 large carrot, chopped

1 celery stalk, cut into pieces

4 thyme sprigs

1 bay leaf

7 cups Chicken bone broth or low-sodium chicken stock

1 tbsp. finely grated ginger

1 zucchini, cut into cubes

500 g/17.6 oz Kent pumpkin, cut into cubes

450 g/15.8 oz shredded poached chicken

200 g/7 oz silverbeet shredded

freshly ground black pepper

Method:

Add the oil into a stockpot over medium heat and add the onion, garlic, carrot, celery, thyme and bay leaf. Cook, stirring occasionally, for 6 minutes until the vegetables are soft.

Pour the broth/stock into the pot and bring to the boil, then reduce the heat to low and simmer for 20 minutes.

Add the ginger, zucchini and pumpkin to the pot and cook for a further 15 minutes. Add the poached chicken and silverbeet and simmer for another few minutes until the silverbeet is cooked.

Season the soup with pepper and sprinkle on the parsley.

Chicken Broth

Ingredients:

1 kg/35 oz chicken frames/bones

4 chicken feet (optional)

2 tbsps. apple cider vinegar

1 large onion, roughly chopped

2 carrots. roughly chopped

3 celery stalks, roughly chopped

2 leeks, white part only, roughly chopped

1 garlic bulb, cut in half horizontally

1 tbsp. black peppercorns, lightly crushed

2 bay leaves

2 large handfuls of flat-leaf parsley stalks

Method:

Place the chicken pieces in a stockpot, add 5 L/169 fl oz of cold water, the vinegar, onion, carrot, celery, peppercorns and bay leaves and let sit for 30 mins.

Place the pot over medium-high heat and bring to the boil and then reduce the heat to low and simmer for anywhere up to 12 hours or longer.

Strain the broth into an airtight container and place refrigerate. The following day you will notice a layer of fat the top, this can be discarded. You'll also note the broths become a jelly which is the gelatine from the bones.

The broth can be stored in the fridge for 3-4 days or frozen for up to 3 months.

Note that while there are claims that bone broth is great for digestive health and overall nutrition, this recipe will be high in protein, phosphorus and potassium. Mostly this would be used as an ingredient in other recipes as a fresh, low-sodium alternative to store bought stocks.

Cream of Cauliflower Soup

Ingredients:

1 tbsp. olive oil

1 brown onion, finely chopped

2 garlic cloves, crushed

2 tsp ground coriander

1 tsp ground cumin

1/4 tsp chilli flakes

750g/26 oz cauliflower, trimmed, cut into florets

2 cups low sodium vegetable stock

2 cups water

1/4 cup pouring cream or creme fraiche

Method:

Heat oil in a saucepan over medium heat. Add onion and garlic. Cook, stirring, for 6 to 7 minutes or until very soft.

Add coriander, cumin and chilli flakes. Increase heat to high. Cook, stirring, for 2 minutes. Add cauliflower, stock and water. Cover. Bring to the boil. Reduce heat to low. Simmer, partially covered, for 30 minutes or until cauliflower is tender. Set aside for 20 minutes.

Blend soup in batches until smooth. Return to saucepan. Stir in cream. Stir over low heat until hot. Season with salt and pepper.

Cauliflower Purée with Thyme

Ingredients:

1 head cauliflower, cut into 1/2-inch pieces

1 cup chicken broth

1 tsp salt, plus more to taste

3 tbsps. unsalted butter, cut into chunks

1 tsp chopped fresh thyme

Freshly ground black pepper, to taste

Method:

In a large pot, bring the chicken broth and salt to a boil.

Add the cauliflower; bring back to a boil. Cover, reduce the heat to low and steam for 20 minutes, or until cauliflower is very tender.

Use a slotted spoon to transfer the cauliflower to a food processor.

Add 3 tablespoons of chicken broth from the pot, along with the butter.

Process until smooth. Taste and season with freshly ground pepper. Add thyme and process until just combined.

Mediterranean Roasted Red Pepper Soup

Ingredients:

2 tbsps. olive oil

6 garlic cloves, minced

1 tsp paprika

1/2 cup lentils, sorted and rinsed

3 fresh red peppers, roasted

1 can (28 oz) diced tomatoes

2 cups chicken broth or water

1/2 cup non-fat milk powder

1 tbsp. red wine vinegar

1/4 cup cashews or almonds, toasted

Method:

Heat olive oil, add onions and cook slowly, stirring occasionally until onions are very soft and caramelized.

Add garlic and paprika, cook for 2 minutes.

Add lentils, peppers, tomatoes, and 1 cup broth.

Bring to boil, reduce heat to maintain a steady simmer, cover, and cook lentils until they are soft (about 30 min).

In several batches, whirl soup in blender or food processor until very smooth.

Add milk powder and vinegar to the last batch. Stir together.

Season with more vinegar if needs more taste and add in a little more broth if soup seems too thick.

Serve topped with a sparkle of almonds and a drizzle of oil if you like.

Chicken Veg Noodle Soup

Ingredients:

2 tbsps. vegetable oil

2 chicken breasts

1 onion, chopped

3-4 carrots, chopped

2 celery stalks with leaves

6 cups chicken broth or low-sodium chicken stock

1 cup frozen peas

1 cup frozen corn

2 tbsps. lime juice

1 bay leaf

2 tbsps. parsley

1/2 tsp salt

1/4 tsp pepper

1 cup egg noodles

Method:

In the pressure cooker, heat 1 tbsp. oil over medium heat. Add chicken and cook for 5 minutes, or until browned on both sides. Remove chicken breasts from the pot and dice into small pieces. Set aside.

Add 1 tbsp. oil, onions, carrots and celery to the pot. Cook for around 2 minutes, stirring occasionally.

Add the broth, peas, corn, lime juice, bay leaf, parsley and season with salt and pepper. Next, add the noodles.

Secure the lid and bring to pressure on high heat. Reduce heat to the lowest level while maintaining pressure. Cook for 8 minutes. Add pepper to taste.

Root Vegetable Soup

Ingredients:

6 tbsps. unsalted butter

1 large onion, chopped

2 to 3 celery stalks, diced

3 garlic cloves, finely chopped

3 rosemary or thyme branches

2 bay leaves

3 1/2 pounds (1.5 kg) mixed root vegetables (carrot, parsnip, celery root, turnip, rutabaga, sweet or regular potato), peeled and cut into 1-inch (2.5 cm) chunks

1/2 tsp black pepper, more as needed

Juice of 1/2 lemon, more for serving

Olive oil

Grated Parmesan, optional

Method:

Par-boil any potatoes and throw away the water. This reduces their potassium content.

Melt butter in a large, heavy-bottomed pot. Stir in onion and celery. Cook, stirring occasionally, until vegetables are tender, about 10 minutes. Stir in garlic, rosemary and bay leaves; cook 1 minute more.

Add root vegetables, 8 cups water, salt and pepper. Bring to a boil; reduce heat to medium and simmer, covered, until vegetables are tender, 25 to 35 minutes.

Remove and discard rosemary branches and bay leaves. Using a blender, purée the soup until smooth. If the soup is too thick, add a little water and add lemon juice to taste.

Serve into bowls and top with a drizzle of olive oil, grated parmesan and a dash of lemon juice.

Simple Chicken Soup

Ingredients:

4 chicken thigh cutlets, skinned, excess fat trimmed

1 large brown onion, halved, finely chopped

1 large carrot, peeled, finely chopped

1 celery stick, trimmed, finely chopped

2 large garlic cloves, finely chopped

2 tablespoons finely chopped fresh continental parsley stems

6 sprigs fresh thyme, leaves picked

8 cups water

1/2 tsp whole black peppercorns

1/4 cup finely chopped fresh continental parsley, extra

Method:

Combine chicken, onion, carrot, celery, garlic, parsley, thyme, water and peppercorns in a large saucepan over medium-high heat. Bring to the boil. Reduce heat to low and cook, covered, for 40 minutes or until vegetables are very tender.

Use tongs to transfer the chicken to a clean work surface. Hold with tongs and cut the chicken meat from the bones. Discard bones. Tear the chicken meat and add to the soup.

Ladle soup among serving bowls. Sprinkle with extra parsley and serve immediately.

Thai Style Pumpkin Soup

Ingredients:

25g/.88 oz Butter

100 g/3.5 oz Brown onion, diced

600 g/21 oz Butternut pumpkin, peeled and diced

700 ml/23.6 fl oz chicken broth or low-sodium chicken stock

1 tsp Sugar

1 tsp fresh Ginger, finely chopped

1/4 bunch Coriander, chopped

1/2 stem Lemon-grass

1 tsp Fresh chilli, finely chopped

150 ml/5 fl oz Coconut milk

Sour cream, and coriander sprig to garnish

Method:

Place the butter into a soup pot/stock pot, add the diced onions and pumpkin and allow to cook without browning over moderate heat.

Add the chicken stock/broth, sugar, ginger, coriander, lemon-grass, and chilli.

Cook until all the vegetables are soft, approximately one-hour.

Remove the lemon-grass and purée the soup in a blender and return to the pot, bring to the boil, add the coconut milk and pepper and a little more stock or water to reach the desired puree-like consistency.

Serve and garnish with sour cream and coriander.

Cauliflower Apple Soup

1 head cauliflower, chopped into small florets

1 cup yellow onion, diced

1 cup apple, diced

2 cloves garlic, minced

1 teaspoon sage

1 teaspoon thyme

1 teaspoon rosemary

1/2 teaspoon ground black pepper

6 cups low-sodium chicken stock or chicken bone broth

Add the vegetables, dry spices, and chicken stock into a large sauce pan and bring to a boil.

Reduce heat and simmer for approximately 30 minutes or until the vegetables have softened.

With a hand blender, puree the soup until smooth.

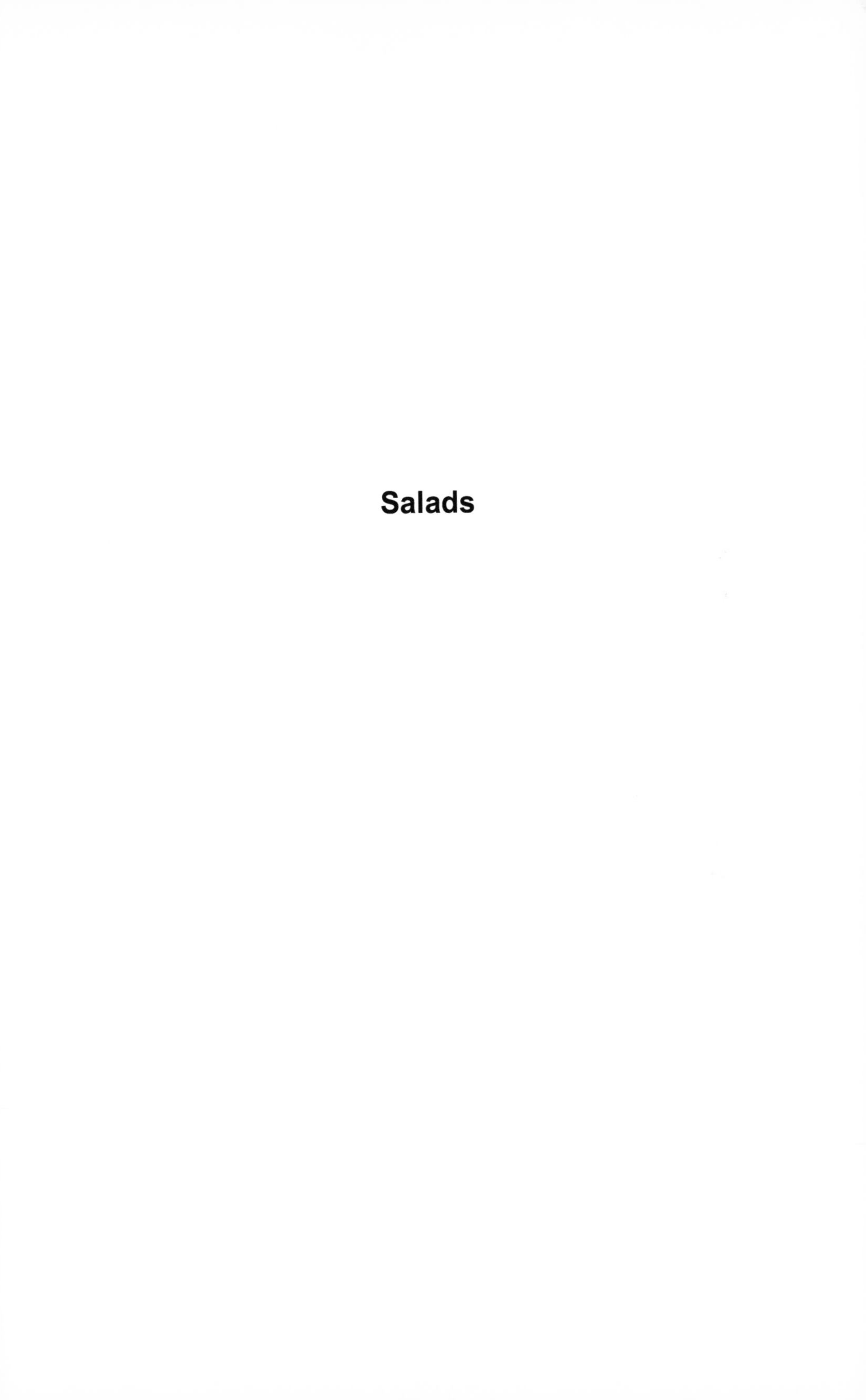

Salads

Tuna Salad

Ingredients:

A large tin of tuna

1 finely chopped shallot (scallion)

2 finely chopped radishes

1 piece of celery finely chopped

1 tbsp. of mild mustard

1 tbsp. of flax seed oil

a pinch of cayenne pepper.

Method:

Mix the tuna with all other ingredients in a medium sized bowl.

Asparagus Balsamic Salad

Ingredients:

1/3 cup balsamic vinegar

3 tbsps. olive oil

1 tbsp. Dijon mustard

1 tsp. marjoram

1 tsp minced garlic

900 g/2 pounds asparagus

1 small red bell pepper (capsicum), diced

1/3 cup chopped pecans, toasted

Method:

Boil vinegar in a small saucepan over medium heat until reduced by half, about 3 minutes. Pour vinegar into large bowl and whisk in oil, mustard, marjoram and garlic. Season with pepper.

Cut the tough ends off the asparagus and slice into 1 inch pieces. Bring a large pot of water to the boil and drop in the asparagus and cook until tender, about 4 minutes. Drain and rinse.

Add asparagus and bell pepper (capsicum) to the dressing and toss. Sprinkle with pecans and serve.

Carrot Salad

Ingredients:

500 g/17 oz carrots

2-3 gherkins

1 onion

3 tbsps. of sunflower seeds

4 tbsps. of flax seed oil

4 tbsps. of lemon juice

2 tbsps. mineral water

a handful of parsley

Method:

Finely grate the carrots.

Slice the gherkins.

Mix the carrot, gherkin, finely chopped onion and sunflower seeds.

Mix the oil, mineral water and lemon juice and add to the salad.

Stand for 20 minutes and let the flavours develop.

Top with parsley.

Herb Cucumber Salad

Ingredients:

2 large cucumbers

3 tbsps. extra-virgin olive oil

1/2 lemon, juiced

1 tbsp. apple cider vinegar

1 tsp dijon mustard

2 tbsps. chopped fresh dill

2 tbsps. chopped fresh parsley

1 tbsp. chopped fresh mint

1/4 tsp garlic granules

Pinch of red pepper flakes

Method:

Slice cucumbers.

In a bowl combine oil, vinegar, mustard, fresh herbs, garlic, and red pepper flakes.

Pour mixture over cucumbers and toss to coat evenly. Let sit for 10 minutes.

Serve immediately.

Cucumber and Mint Salad

Ingredients:

4 Lebanese cucumbers

2 green shallots (scallions), ends trimmed, thinly sliced

1/4 cup fresh coriander leaves

1/2 cup fresh mint leaves

1/4 cup yoghurt

1 garlic clove, crushed

1 tbsp. fresh lime juice

2 tsp water

1 tsp finely grated lime rind

Method:

Trim the ends of the cucumbers, cut in half lengthways, remove the seeds and slice thinly and diagonally.

Combine the cucumber, shallot, coriander and mint in a medium bowl. Cover and place in the fridge.

Combine the yoghurt, garlic, lime juice, water and lime rind and season with pepper.

Cover and place in the fridge for 20 minutes.

Place the cucumber mixture on a serving platter and drizzle over the yoghurt dressing.

Serve immediately.

Radish Cucumber Salad

Ingredients:

2 cups sliced radishes

1 cup sliced red onion

1 cup seeded and sliced cucumber

1/2 cup extra virgin olive oil

2 tbsps. white wine vinegar

1/2 tsp white sugar

1 clove garlic, minced

1 tsp chopped fresh dill

Method:

Toss radishes with a little of the vinegar; let stand for about 10 minutes. Drain any liquid and transfer radishes to a large bowl. Add red onion and cucumber slices.

Whisk olive oil, vinegar, sugar, garlic, and dill in a small bowl until well mixed; pour over vegetables and toss to combine. Cover and refrigerate for at least 1 hour before serving.

Carrot Salad

Ingredients:

750g/24 oz carrots, cut into thick slices

Dressing:

1 clove garlic, crushed

1/2 tsp paprika

1/2 tsp cumin

1/2 tsp chilli powder (optional)

2 tbsps. lemon juice

2 tbsps. olive oil

pinch sugar

Garnish:

Coriander or parsley leaves, chopped

Method:

Boil carrots slices in until tender, about 10-15 minutes, then drain.

Combine all the dressing ingredients, then pour over the carrots straight away.

Garnish with coriander or parsley leaves.

Homemade Coleslaw

Ingredients:

1/2 cup white wine vinegar

2 tbsps. sugar

1/2 tsp. freshly ground black pepper

1 small head green cabbage, halved, cored, thinly sliced

1 large carrot, peeled, shredded

1/4 cup greek yoghurt

1/4 cup mayonnaise

1 1/2 tbsps. Dijon mustard

4 shallots (scallions), finely chopped

Method:

In a large bowl, stir the vinegar, sugar, and pepper until the sugar dissolves. Add the cabbage and carrots and toss to thoroughly coat with the dressing. Cover and refrigerate for 30 minutes.

In a small bowl, stir the yoghurt, mayonnaise, and mustard to blend. Drizzle the mayonnaise dressing over the cabbage mixture and toss to combine thoroughly. Mix in the spring onions and serve.

Tabbouleh

Ingredients:

1 cup Bulgur wheat

1 cup Warm water

1 Tomato, peeled & chopped

1/2 Med. cucumber, seeded & chopped

1/2 cup Snipped parsley

2 tbsps. Green onion (scallion/spring onion), finely chopped

1 tbsp. Fresh mint, finely chopped

1/8 tsp Pepper

3 tbsps. Olive oil

3 tbsps. Lemon juice

Method:

In a bowl, combine bulgur and warm water.

Let stand 1/2 hour.

Stir in tomato, cucumber, parsley, green onion, mint, and pepper.

Combine oil and lemon juice.

Toss with the bulgur mixture.

Cover and chill.

Serve in a lettuce-lined bowl with yoghurt, if desired.

Sesame Pasta Salad

Ingredients:

1 tbsp. Sesame seeds

1/3 of a cup (16 oz/450gm) package Penne pasta

1/2 of pepper Red bell pepper (capsicum), sliced thinly

1/4 of small head Green cabbage, shredded

3 tbsps. Vegetable oil

2 tbsps. low salt soy sauce

2 tbsps. Rice vinegar

1/2 tsp Sesame oil

1 tbsp. Granulated sugar

1/4 tsp Ground ginger

1/8 tsp Ground black pepper

2 tbsps. Fresh cilantro (coriander), chopped

2 tbsps. Green onion (spring onions/scallion), chopped

Method:

Heat skillet (frying pan) over medium-high heat. Add sesame seeds, and cook stirring frequently until lightly toasted. Remove from heat, and set aside.

Bring a large pot of water to a boil. Add pasta, and cook for 8-10 minutes, or until al dente (still slightly firm). Drain pasta, and rinse under cold water until cool.

Transfer to a large bowl. Add sliced red bell pepper (capsicum) and shredded cabbage to the pasta.

In a bottle, combine vegetable oil, soy sauce, vinegar, sesame oil, sugar, sesame seeds, ginger, and pepper. Shake well.

Pour sesame dressing over pasta, and toss to coat evenly. Gently mix in cilantro, and green onions.

Kale and Apple Coleslaw

Ingredients:

For the dressing:

3 tbsps. cider vinegar

2 tbsps. honey

2 tsps. Dijon mustard

1 1/2 tsps. poppy seeds

Freshly ground black pepper

3 tbsps. vegetable oil

1/3 cup small-dice red onion (about 1/4 medium onion)

For the coleslaw:

1 pound flat-leaf kale (about 2 bunches)

2 medium Granny Smith or Fuji apples, or 1 of each

Combine the vinegar, honey, mustard, pepper, and poppy seeds in a bowl and whisk while slowly adding the oil. Once combined, stir in the onion.

Cut out and discard the tough stems of the kale. Slice crosswise into 1/4-inch ribbons, and add to the bowl with the dressing.

Cut the apples into 1-1/2-inch-long matchsticks, and add to the bowl.

Toss to combine. Let the coleslaw sit for at least 15 minutes at room temperature and up to 1 day in the refrigerator for the flavours to meld.

Toss again before serving.

Simple Kale Salad

Ingredients:

1/2 cup pecans

250gm/9 oz kale

4 to 5 medium radishes, thinly sliced

1/2 cup dried sultanas or dried cranberries

1 medium Granny Smith apple

Dressing:

3 tbsps. olive oil

1 1/2 tbsps. apple cider vinegar (or white wine vinegar)

1 tbsp. mustard

2 tsps. honey

freshly ground pepper, to taste

Method:

Toast the pecans for about 5 to 10 minutes, until golden then set aside to cool.

Remove the stems from the kale and chop. You could lightly sear the kale in a pan with some water to soften, or scrunch it up with your hands to soften and bring out more flavor.

Coarsely chop the pecans.

Chop the apple into small, bite-sized pieces.

In a small bowl, whisk the dressing ingredients together.

Add everything into a salad bowl and the pour the dressing over the salad.

Traditional Polish Sauerkraut Salad

Ingredients:

300g/10oz sauerkraut

1 medium red onion

2 sweet apples

2 medium carrots

ground black pepper to taste

1 tsp of sugar

3-4 tbsps. of olive oil

Method:

Chop onion finely, grate apples and carrots.

Mix all the ingredients together put aside for min 20 minutes before serving.

Creamy Potato Salad with Herbs

Ingredients:

3kg/6.6 pounds desiree potatoes

250g/8.8 oz sour cream (or greek yoghurt)

190g/6.7 oz mayonnaise

1/4 cup coarsely chopped fresh dill

1/4 cup coarsely chopped fresh continental parsley

1 garlic clove, crushed

2 tbsps. finely chopped fresh mint

1 tbsp. Dijon mustard

1 tbsp. fresh lemon juice

freshly ground black pepper to taste

4 green shallots (spring onion/green onion), ends trimmed, thinly sliced

Method:

Place the potatoes in a large saucepan and cover with plenty of cold water. Bring to the boil over high heat and cook for 15-20 minutes or until tender. Drain and set aside for 15 minutes to cool slightly. Cut into halves or quarters.

Use a fork to whisk together the sour cream, mayonnaise, dill, parsley, garlic, mint, mustard and lemon juice in a large bowl until well combined. Taste and season with pepper.

Place the potatoes and green shallot in a large serving bowl. Spoon dressing over the potato mixture and gently toss until potatoes are well coated in dressing. Serve immediately.

Potato Salad

Ingredients:

1.6 kg/3.5 pound desiree potatoes, quartered

1/4 cup sugar, divided

6 tbsps. rice wine vinegar, divided

3 sticks celery, finely diced

1 medium red onion, finely diced

4 spring onions (green onion/scallion), only use the green stem, thinly sliced

1 tbsp. dried parsley

1/4 cup chopped sweet spiced gherkins

2 tbsps. mustard

3/4 cup mayonnaise

3/4 cup sour cream

2 tbsps. grated parmesan

Fresh ground black pepper

Method:

Add potatoes to a large saucepan with 2 L (67 fl oz) of water, and 2 tbsps. sugar, and 2 tbsps. vinegar. Bring to a boil over high heat.

Reduce to simmer, and cook, stirring occasionally, until potatoes are tender, about 10 minutes.

Drain potatoes and spreading them out and sprinkling with 2 tbsps. vinegar. Allow to cool to room temperature, about thirty minutes.

Combine remaining sugar, remaining vinegar, celery, onion, spring onion, parsley, pickles, mustard, parmesan, sour cream and mayonnaise in large bowl. Stir to combine. Fold in potatoes.

Season to taste with pepper. Cover and refrigerate for an hour before serving.

Keeps for up to three days in fridge.

Smoked Salmon Salad with Caper Vinaigrette

Ingredients:

3 cups baby spinach leaves

1/3 cup shelled chopped walnuts

1/2 cup shredded smoked salmon

caper vinaigrette (recipe below)

fresh cracked black pepper

Caper Vinaigrette Recipe:

3/4 cup olive oil

1/4 cup white wine vinegar

1 clove garlic, minced

1 tbsp. minced shallots (green onion/spring onion)

1 tbsp. Dijon mustard

2 tsps. non-pareil capers, rinsed

fresh cracked pepper and kosher salt

Method:

In a bowl combine the spinach, walnuts and salmon and set aside.

In a bowl combine the oil, vinegar, garlic, onions, mustard, capers, and pepper to taste. Set aside at room temperature for 30 minutes.

When ready, whisk the dressing and spoon a few tbsp over the salad as desired, toss and serve.

Baby Spinach with Radishes and Lemon Caper Dressing

Ingredients:

Salad:

450 g/1 pound baby spinach

2 fresh cucumbers

A bunch of radishes

Dressing:

2 tsp capers, drained and rinsed

4 tbsps. olive oil

1 small clove garlic, finely minced

2 tbsps. lemon juice

1 tsp lemon zest

Method:

Rinse the capers with cold water. Roughly chop the garlic and add to a food processor with the capers, oil, lemon juice and zest, and blend till smooth.

Thinly slice the cucumbers and radishes. Tear, or roughly chop the baby spinach into smaller pieces.

Bring everything together and toss to combine.

Kidney Bean Salad

Ingredients:

200gm of kidney beans (cooked - see recipe below)

1/2 cucumber, finely diced

1 cup chopped coriander

1 stick chopped celery

1 cup kale, lightly seared, chopped

2 small radish, Sliced

1/2 red onion finely sliced

For the dressing:

3 tbsps. lime juice

2 tbsp. olive oil

1 tsp mustard

1 clove of garlic

1 tsp of ground cumin

1/2 tsp of oregano

A pinch of pepper to taste

Method:

So simple, throw everything together in a big bowl, then mix the dressing ingredients and drizzle that over the top.

Note: the kale can be seared a little in a pan with a little water, just to soften it, then let it cool before adding with the other ingredients, you could also cut out the hard stems if they are undesirable.

Kidney Beans

Ingredients:

1/2 cup dried Kidney Beans

2 cloves garlic

1 bay leaf

1/2 small onion

Method:

Wash beans and soak overnight in 4 cups of water (use a jar that has some headroom as the beans will grow as the soak up the water).

Rinse the soaked beans and add to the pressure cooker with 3 to 1 ratio of water. Add garlic, bay leaf and onion. Cook for 8 minutes and allow pressure cooker to cool down naturally.

For stovetop, boil the beans for ten minutes to destroy any toxins, then simmer until soft (about 45-60 minutes)

Allow to cool and store in a sealed container in their cooking juices. Store for no more than 3 days.

Poached Chicken Salad

Ingredients:

2 (400g/14 oz) chicken breast fillets

3/4 cup mayonnaise

1/4 cup Greek Yoghurt

1 tbsp. mango chutney

1 tsp curry powder

2 tbsps. finely chopped fresh chives

2 baby cos lettuce hearts, leaves separated

2 medium nectarines, cut into wedges

2 Lebanese cucumbers, finely chopped

1/4 cup flaked almonds, toasted

Method:

Place chicken in a large saucepan. Cover with cold water. Bring to the boil over medium heat. Reduce heat to low. Cover. Simmer for 5 to 7 minutes or until almost cooked through. Remove from heat. Stand for 5 minutes. Remove chicken from pan. Cool. Slice.

Combine mayonnaise, yoghurt, chutney, curry powder and chives in a bowl.

Arrange lettuce leaves, nectarine, cucumber and chicken on a large plate. Drizzle with dressing. Sprinkle with almonds. Serve.

Smoked Salmon Salad

Ingredients:

3 cups baby spinach leaves

1/3 cup honey walnuts

1/2 cup shredded smoked salmon

Caper Vinaigrette Recipe:

3/4 cup (180 ml/6 oz) olive oil

1/4 cup (60 ml/2 oz) white wine vinegar

1 clove garlic, minced

1 tbsp. minced shallots

1 tbsp. mustard

2 tsps. capers, rinsed

fresh cracked pepper

Method:

Some people like spinach leaves as they are, some people like to scrunch them a little to make them softer to eat and release more flavor. Your choice. In a bowl combine spinach, walnuts and salmon.

In another bowl combine all ingredients for caper vinaigrette. Allow to sit at room temperature for 30 minutes.

Give the dressing a quick whisk and drizzle a few tablespoons over the salad. Toss to combine. Sprinkle fresh cracked pepper over the top and serve.

Honey Walnuts:

Set a pan on low and add 1 tbsp. of butter, add 1 cup walnuts and let the walnuts warm, a few minutes. Note the walnuts only need to heat up and not toast or brown. Once warm, with a spoon drizzle over 2 tbsps. of honey, and optionally sprinkle over some sesame seeds. Keep it warming for a minute or two to melt the honey over the walnut, stirring occasionally. Allow to cool completely then break up and store in an airtight container.

Warm Mediterranean Chicken Salad

Ingredients:

2 red capsicums (bell peppers), trimmed, seeded and cut into 5 cm pieces

8 small truss tomatoes, halved

4 Japanese eggplants (aubergines), trimmed and halved lengthways

3 zucchini (courgettes), trimmed and thickly sliced on the diagonal

1 tbsp. olive oil

1 1/2 tsps. smoked paprika

olive oil spray

800 g/1.7 lb skinless chicken thigh fillets, trimmed of fat

2-3 tbsps. balsamic vinegar, or to taste

small handful basil leaves (optional)

1 head radicchio, tough outer leaves discarded, torn

Method:

Preheat the oven to 180C (356F).

Place the capsicum (bell peppers), tomato, eggplant, zucchini(courgettes), olive oil and paprika in a large roasting tin and toss to combine well. Spray another large roasting tin with olive oil, add the chicken and toss to coat. Roast the vegetables and the chicken for 35 minutes or until cooked through. Transfer the vegetables to a bowl.

Transfer the chicken to a board, reserving the cooking juices. When cool enough to handle, cut the chicken into 1 cm thick slices and add to the vegetables in the bowl along with the balsamic vinegar, reserved cooking juices, basil (if using) and radicchio (if using).

Season to taste and toss to combine well, then divide among plates and serve immediately.

Spinach, Pear and Walnut salad

Ingredients:

40 g/1.4 oz walnuts

1 tbsp. extra virgin olive oil

1 tbsp. balsamic vinegar

150 g/5.3 oz baby spinach leaves

1 pear, thinly sliced

Method:

Preheat the oven to 180C (356F) and line a baking tray with baking paper. Spread out the walnuts on the prepared tray and toast them in the oven for 10 minutes or until golden brown and fragrant. Remove from the oven and allow to cool, then roughly chop.

Meanwhile, make a dressing by combining the olive oil and vinegar in a screw-top jar. Shake well to combine.

In a large bowl, gently toss together the spinach leaves, pear slices and dressing. Arrange on serving plates and scatter the walnuts over the top.

Broccoli and Almond Salad

Ingredients:
1 small head broccoli, cut into florets and lightly steamed or blanched

1 bunch spring onions (scallions), thinly sliced

1 small head butter lettuce, washed and torn into pieces

1 bunch radishes, washed and sliced into strips

1 small red (Spanish) onion, thinly sliced

1 cup almonds, cut into slivers or coarsely chopped

Tahini dressing

Method:
Add all the vegetables to a large bowl and gently toss until combined.

Sprinkle the almonds over the top or serve them separately in a bowl.

Pour the tahini dressing over the salad just before serving.

Beetroot and Pistachio Salad

Ingredients:
6 large beetroots (beets), leaves removed just above the stalk and cut in half

1 small bunch chives, finely chopped

1 small bunch lemon thyme, leaves removed from the woody stalk and chopped

5 or 6 spring onions (scallions), finely sliced including the green part

1 small lettuce, to serve

1 cup salted pistachio nuts, shelled and coarsely chopped, to serve

Simple Salad Dressing:

zest and juice from 1 lime

1/4 cup olive oil

1 small clove garlic, peeled

sea salt and freshly ground black pepper, to taste

Method:
Boil the beetroot in water for 30 minutes or until soft. They are cooked when a sharp knife slides easily into the vegetable.

Toss the herbs and spring onions in a large bowl.

When the beetroots are cooked, allow them to cool just a little, retaining some heat to release the oils in the herbs.

Cut off the beetroot tops, peel the skin and then cut them in half again so you are working with a quarter of a beetroot. Slice the quarters into slivers and toss with the herbs and spring onions. Arrange on the lettuce leaves.

To make the dressing, place all the ingredients in a blender and mix until well combined.

Pour the dressing over the salad, sprinkle with the pistachios and enjoy the gorgeous colours and flavours!

Variation:

Use 1/2 cup freshly chopped coriander (cilantro) for a different flavour and top with walnuts instead of pistachios.

Simple Cucumber Salad

Method:

Peel the cucumber and cut lengthwise to give two halves. Scoop out the seeds with a spoon.

Cut the cucumber into thin slices and arrange in a suitable bowl.

Add a dill infused Vinaigrette, mix through and garnish with a sprig of fresh dill.

Waldorf Salad

Ingredients:
500 g/17.6 oz Apples, julienne

500 g/17.6 oz Celery, julienne

3 tbsps. Lemon juice

200 g/7 oz Walnuts, chopped

1 1/2 cups Mayonnaise

3/4 cup Cream

Method:
Place the julienne of apple and celery into a stainless-steel bowl and mix with the lemon juice to prevent the apples from browning.

Mix the mayonnaise and cream together and add to the salad with the chopped walnuts and mix together well.

Adjust the seasoning and dress neatly in a salad bowl. Garnish with walnut pieces scattered on top.

Greek Salad

Ingredients:
2 Continental cucumber

2 Onion, sliced into thin rings

2 Ripe tomatoes, cut in wedges

150 g/5.2 oz Black Greek olives

2-3 leaves Iceberg lettuce

2-3 leaves Cos lettuce

1/4 bunch Oregano fresh chopped

3 tbsps. Lemon juice

1/2 cup Olive oil

200 g/7 oz Fetta cheese, 2 cm cubes

Pepper to taste

Method:
Wash the lettuce in cold water. drain well and tear into bite-sized pieces.

Peel the cucumber and cut into chunky slices.

Combine the cucumber, onion rings, tomato wedges, olives and chopped oregano together with the lettuce and mix well. Add the fetta on top of the salad.

Make a vinaigrette with the lemon juice, olive oil, pepper and dress the salad.

Caesar Salad

Ingredients:
20 leaves Cos lettuce

2 cloves Garlic

1/2 cup Olive oil

200 g/7 oz White bread

3 Eggs

3/4 cup Olive oil

1/3 cup Lemon juice

Black pepper, finely ground to taste

30 g/1 oz Anchovy fillets

100 g/3.5 oz Parmesan, shaved

Method:
Wash the lettuce in cold water, tear into bite-sized pieces and leave to drain well.

Remove the crust from the bread and evenly cut into 1 cm cubes.

Heat the peeled garlic cloves and half the olive oil gently in a frying pan. Add the bread and cook while continually turning until the croutons are crisp and golden brown.

Drain the croutons on absorbent paper,

Cut the anchovy fillets into small pieces, and shave the Parmesan using a vegetable peeler or a slicer. Set these aside for further use.

Coddle the eggs by placing them into boiling water for one minute.

Break the eggs into a bowl. add the remaining olive oil, lemon juice and pepper and mix well.

To serve, place the lettuce in a bowl and toss with the coddled egg dressing. Scatter the croutons and anchovy on top and finish with the shaved Parmesan.

Serve.

Nicoise Salad

Ingredients:
200 g/7 oz Washed potatoes, chats

150g/5.2 oz Green beans, trimmed

3 Tomatoes, peeled

100 g/3.5 oz Tinned tuna, flaked and drained

1/3 cup Wine vinegar

3/4 cup Olive oil

2 cloves Garlic, crushed

Pepper and salt to taste

80 g/2.8 oz Black olives

5 Anchovy fillets

30 g/1 oz Capers

5 leaves Butter lettuce, washed,

25 g/.9 oz Parsley, chopped

Method:
Boil the potatoes in their skins in salted water, drain and allow to cool. Peel the potatoes and cut them into 1.5 cm cubes.

Trim, blanch and refresh and drain the beans. Cut each peeled tomato into 8 wedges.

Make a garlic dressing using the olive oil, vinegar, pepper and salt.

To serve, lay the washed lettuce on a platter, arrange a layer of

potato, then green beans,
then tuna and finish with tomato wedges.

Moisten with garlic dressing and dress with olives, capers and anchovy fillets.

Sprinkle with chopped parsley and serve.

Salad Dressings

Balsamic Syrup

Ingredients:

1/2 cup (120 ml/4 fl oz) balsamic vinegar

1/2 cup brown sugar

Method:

Combine the brown sugar and balsamic vinegar in a small pan and stir constantly while slowly bringing to the boil. Reduce the heat and allow the mixture to simmer for 5 minutes until thickened.

Classic Vinaigrette

Ingredients:

1 1/2 tbsps. red wine vinegar

1 tbsp. chopped shallots

1 tbsp. Dijon mustard

1/8 tsp pepper

3 tbsps. extra-virgin olive oil

Method:

Combine vinegar, shallots, salt, Dijon mustard, and pepper. Gradually add olive oil, stirring until incorporated.

Sweet Soy Dressing

Ingredients:

2 tbsp. soy sauce (salt reduced)

1 tbsp. fresh lemon juice

3 tbsp. brown sugar

1 tbsp. finely chopped Vietnamese mint, optional

Method:

Combine lemon juice, soy, sugar and mint in a bottle and shake well. This dressing matches well with Asian greens and salads.

Honey Dressing

Ingredients:

1/4 cup olive oil

1 tbsp. red wine vinegar

3 tbsp. honey

Fresh cracked pepper

Method:

Combine ingredients in a bottle and shake well. Add pepper to taste. Great for salads, especially warm salads.

Lemon Balsamic

Ingredients:

6 tbsps. extra virgin olive oil

2 tbsps. balsamic vinegar

2 tbsps. honey

1 tbsp. freshly squeezed lemon juice

1/2 tsp black pepper

1/2 tsp garlic

Method:

Combine ingredients in a bowl and whisk until well blended. If refrigerating, whisk again before use.

Italian dressing

Ingredients:
250 ml/8.4 fl oz White wine vinegar

750 ml/25 fl oz Olive oil

1.5 tsp Garlic Powder

1 tbsp. Oregano, chopped

2 tbsps. Parsley, chopped

Pepper to taste

Method:

Combine all ingredients in a bowl and mix well. Mix again before using.

Mustard Vinaigrette

Ingredients:
250 ml/8.4 fl oz White wine vinegar

750 ml/25.3 fl oz Salad Oil

50 g/1.7 fl oz Mustard, French Or Dijon

Pepper to taste

Method:

Mix the vinegar and mustard together add the oil and pepper and mix well.

Mix and stir again before using.

Walnut Herb Vinaigrette

Ingredients:

250 ml/8.4 fl oz Cider vinegar

375 ml/12.6 fl oz Walnut oil

375 ml/12.7 fl oz Peanut oil

1 tbsp. Parsley, chopped

1 tbsp. Chives, chopped

1 tbsp. Chervil, chopped

Pepper to taste

Method:

Season the vinegar with the pepper and gradually whisk in the oils, a little at a time followed by the herbs.

Mix and stir again before using.

Simple Honey Lemon Dressing

Ingredients:
250 ml/8.4 fl oz Honey

250 ml/8.4 fl oz Lemon juice

Method:

Mix honey and lemon juice together until thoroughly combined.

Honey Lemon Dressing with Thyme

Ingredients:

1 tbsp. plus 2 teaspoons fresh lemon juice

1 tsp finely grated lemon zest

1 tbsp. honey

1/2 tsp chopped thyme

1/4 cup extra-virgin olive oil

Freshly ground pepper

Method:

In a small bowl, whisk the lemon juice with the lemon zest, honey and thyme. Whisk in the olive oil and season with salt and pepper.

Honey Lemon Dressing with Basil

Ingredients:

1/4 cup honey

3 tbsps. lemon juice

2 tbsps. vegetable oil

1/2 tsp. dried basil

1/2 tsp. crushed red pepper flakes

Method:

Whisk together all ingredients in small bowl until well blended.

Fruit Salad Dressing

Ingredients:
5 tbsps. Sugar

1 tbsp. Cornflour

2 Eggs

1/2 cup Pineapple juice

1/2 cup Orange juice

1/4 cup Lemon juice

1/2 cup Sour cream

Method:

Mix the sugar and cornflour together in a bowl and add the eggs and beat until the mixture is smooth.

Mix the three fruit juices together in a pan and bring to the boil.

Remove from the heat and gradually beat the boiling liquid into the egg mixture and return to the pan.

Bring to the boil again while stirring constantly. When the mixture thickens, strain it into a

clean bowl and chill in the refrigerator.

Beat the sour cream into the chilled juice mixture.

Rosemary and Mustard Dressing

Ingredients:

1 cup olive oil

1/3 cup lemon juice

2 tsps. freshly chopped rosemary leaves

2 tsps. dry mustard

3 spring onions (scallions)

2 cloves garlic

2 tsps. maple syrup (or honey)

Freshly ground black pepper, to taste

Method:

Place all the ingredients in a powerful blender and blend until the rosemary leaves are finely crushed.

Store the dressing in the refrigerator in an airtight container for about 5 days.

Creamy Tahini Salad Dressing

Ingredients:

1 cup tahini

1 cup water

3 tbsps. lemon juice

1 large clove garlic, peeled

freshly ground black pepper, to taste

2 tsps. dried Italian herbs

Method:

Place all the ingredients in a powerful blender and blend until creamy.

Store the dressing in the refrigerator in an airtight container for about 5 days.

Salad Dressing

Ingredients:

4 tbsps. sesame oil

4 tbsps. flax seed oil

1 tbsp. balsamic vinegar

3 tbsps. rice vinegar

2 tbsps. black currant syrup

Method:

Mix all ingredients. Serve as a dressing with a green salad.

Basil Dressing

Ingredients:

1/4 cup flax oil

1/4 cup water

3 tbsps. lemon juice

2 tbsps. basil

1 tsp garlic

Method:

Combine in blender or food processor and blend.

Lemon-Tarragon Dressing

Ingredients:

1/4 lemon juice

1 tsp Dijon mustard

2 tbsps. flax oil

2 tsp chopped fresh tarragon

Method:

Mix all ingredients.

Red Chilli Mustard Vinegar

Ingredients:

2 tbsps. Dijon mustard

1 tbsp. shallots, chopped

1 tbsp. chilli powder

1/4 cup red wine vinegar

1/2 cup olive oil

Pepper to taste

Method:

Whisk mustard, chilli powder, and vinegar and continue to whisk while adding oil until combined.

Add pepper to taste.

Creamy Basil Vinaigrette Dressing

Ingredients:

1/2 cup Olive oil

1/4 cup Red wine vinegar

1 tbsp. Fresh basil

2 tsp Granulated sugar

1/4 tsp Ground pepper

1 tsp Garlic powder

Method:

Combine all ingredients in a blender.

Buttermilk Herb Ranch Dressing

Ingredients:

1/2 cup mayonnaise

1/2 cup milk

2 tbsps. vinegar

1 tbsp. fresh chives, chopped

1 tbsp. dill

1 tbsp. oregano leaves, chopped

1/4 tsp garlic powder

Method:

In a medium bowl, whisk 1/2 cup each of mayonnaise and milk and 2 tablespoons vinegar.

Then add 1 tablespoon of chopped fresh chives, dill, and oregano leaves with 1/4 teaspoon garlic powder.

Mix together.

Chill at least one hour to allow flavours to develop.

Stir dressing well before serving.

Homemade Mayonnaise

Ingredients:
6 Egg yolks

1/4 cup White vinegar

1 tbsp. French mustard paste

1L/33fl oz Olive Oil

2 tbsps. Lemon juice

Pepper

Method:

Mix the egg yolks, vinegar, mustard, and a pinch of pepper thoroughly with a whisk.

Gradually drizzle the oil into the vinegar mixture while mixing vigorously and continually until an emulsion forms.

Gradually beat in the remaining oil alternately with the lemon juice.

Stabilise the mix by whisking in 1 tbsp. of cold water.

Keep in fridge for 4-5 days.

Homemade Mayonnaise II

Ingredients:
4 egg yolks
2 tsps. Dijon mustard
1 tbsp. apple cider vinegar
1 tbsp. lemon juice
1 1/2 cups olive oil
freshly ground black pepper

Method:
Place the egg yolks, mustard, vinegar, lemon juice into a food processor combine.

With the motor running, slowly pour in the oil and process until the mayonnaise is thick and creamy. Add pepper to taste.

Store in the fridge for 4-5 days.

Homemade Aioli (garlic mayonnaise)

Ingredients:
4 tsp Garlic powder
6 Egg yolks
3 tbsps. White vinegar
1 tbsp. French mustard paste
1L/33fl oz Olive Oil
2 tbsps.

Method:
Add the crushed garlic to the egg yolks and proceed as for the base mayonnaise
recipe above. Use as required.

Sauce Andalouse

Ingredients:
1 1/2 cups Mayonnaise

1/2 cup Tomato purée

1 Red capsicum (bell pepper) diced

Method:

Mix all the ingredients together and correct seasoning.

Tartare sauce

Ingredients:
1/3 cup Mayonnaise

1 tbsp. Capers, chopped

1 tbsp. Gherkins, chopped

1 tsp. Parsley, chopped

Method:
Place all the chopped ingredients into a bowl and add the mayonnaise sauce.

Mix well and use as required.

Tartare Sauce II

Ingredients:

3 tbsps. Mayonnaise

1 tbsp. olive oil

1/2 tbsp. parmesan

1/2 tbsp. dried parsley

1 tsp lemon juice

1/2 tsp finely chopped capers

1 small Pickled Gherkin finely chopped

Method:

Blend it all together, pepper to taste.

Macadamia Mayonnaise

Ingredients:
3/4 cup macadamia nuts

juice of 1 lemon

2 tbsps. olive oil

cold water, as required (about 1/3 cup)

Method:
Add the macadamia nuts, lemon juice and olive oil to a blender and combine until smooth, using some of the cold water if it becomes too thick to move.

Store in an airtight container. This cream keeps for about 5 days in the refrigerator.

Mock Mayonnaise

Ingredients:

1/4 cup water

1/4 tsp garlic powder

1/4 tsp salt

1/4 cup flax seed oil

1/4 cup olive oil

2 tbsps. lemon juice

1/4 tsp cider vinegar

Method:

Combine ingredients in descending order in a blender or food processor. Process until thick and creamy.

Mock Hollandaise

Ingredients:

1/2 cup light mayonnaise

1/2 tsp Dijon mustard

4 tsps. fresh lemon juice, or to taste

2 tbsps. unsalted butter

cayenne pepper, to taste

1 tbsp. Parmesan Cheese (optional)

Method:

Combine all ingredients.

Creamy White Sauce

Ingredients:

1/4 cup mayonnaise

2 tsps. white vinegar

1 tsp fresh lemon juice

1/2 tsp freshly ground black pepper

1/4 tsp salt

1 minced garlic clove

Method:

Combine all ingredients, stirring well.

Almond Herb Pesto

Ingredients:
1 small bunch chives

1 small bunch flat-leaf (Italian) parsley

1 small bunch basil

1 small bunch coriander (cilantro)

1 cup almonds

1 tsp. garlic powder

1/2 cup olive oil

Juice of 1 lemon

Method:
Add all the ingredients to a blender or food processor and pulse until coarsely blended.

Keeps for up to 5 days, refrigerated in an airtight container.

Great with pasta and roast cauliflower.

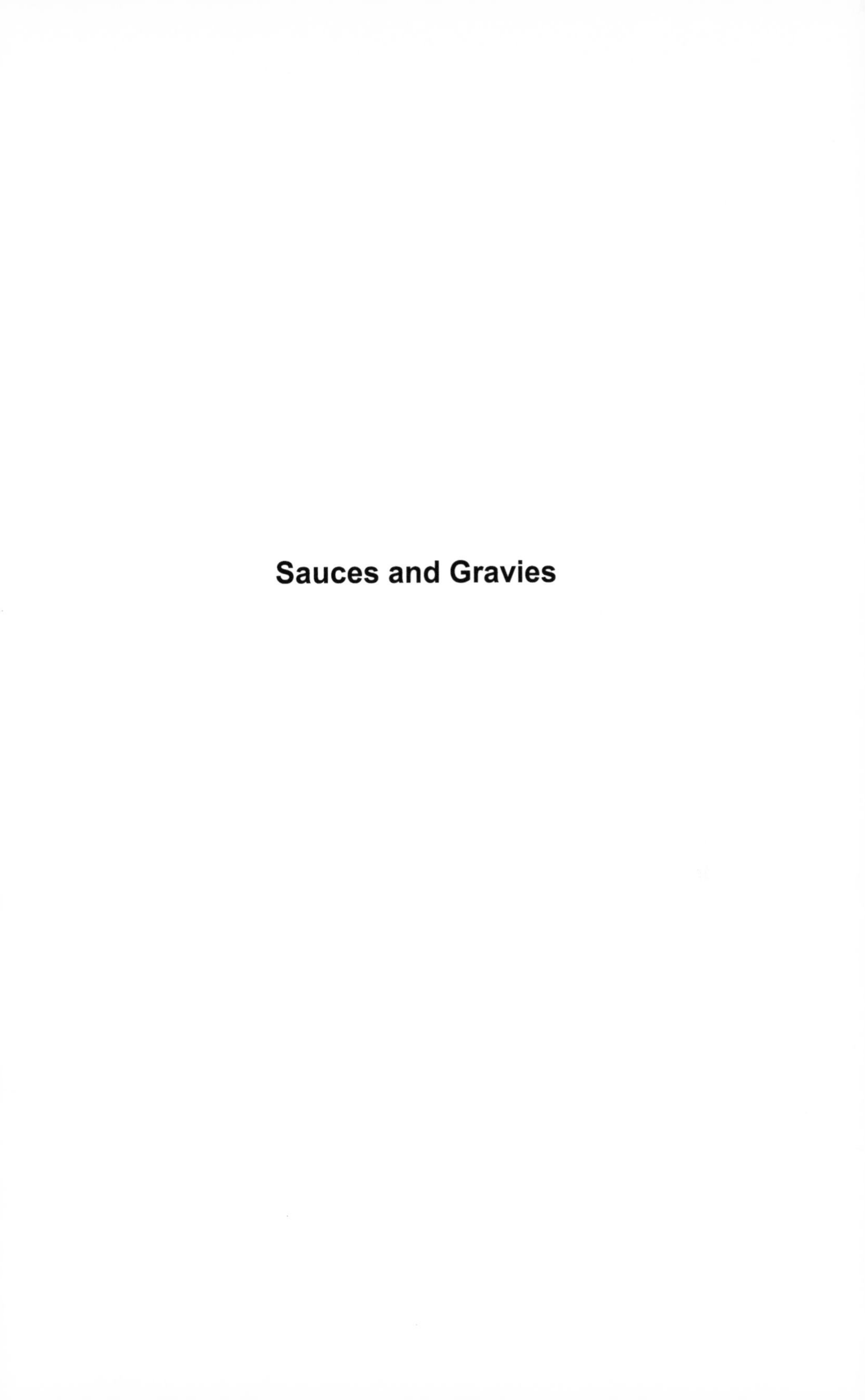

Sauces and Gravies

Garlic Rosemary Sauce

Ingredients:

2 garlic cloves

freshly ground black pepper

2 tbsps. olive oil

2 tbsps. rosemary

2 tbsps. fresh lemon juice

1/2 cup chicken stock

1 tbsp. butter

Method:

Chop garlic. Add garlic, rosemary, lemon juice, and stock to skillet and over high heat, stirring for 1 minute. Whisk in butter.

Great for lamb.

Honey Mustard Sauce

Ingredients:

2 tsps. cornflour

1 1/2 cups Low Sodium Beef Stock

1 tbsp. honey

1 1/2 tbsps. wholegrain mustard

1 green onion, chopped

Method:

Combine the cornflour and 1 tbsp. water in a small bowl and whisk until a smooth paste forms. Place the stock, honey and mustard in a small saucepan over medium heat and cook, stirring, until sauce comes to a simmer. Add the cornflour mixture and green onion, stirring constantly to avoid lumps forming in the sauce. Cook for another 1 minute then set aside.

Can use as dipping sauce or serve with any meat.

Peppercorn Sauce

Ingredients:

2 tbsps. of red wine vinegar

150ml/5 fl oz of chicken stock

2 tsps. of green peppercorns

4 tbsps. of double cream

Method:

Put 2 tbsps. of red wine vinegar into a large, non-stick frying pan and bring to a simmer. Then add 150ml of chicken stock and reduce the mixture by half over a high heat. Add 2 tsps. of green peppercorns, crushing a few of them gently in the pan with the back of a spoon. Season and reduce then stir in 4 tbsps. of double cream. Simmer for one or two minutes until the sauce is slightly thickened.

Faux Béarnaise Sauce

Ingredients:

25g of butter

1 tsp of white wine vinegar

100g/3.5 oz greek yoghurt

1 tsp of Dijon mustard

1/2 tsp of capers

1 shallot (scallion/spring onion)

a small bunch of tarragon

Method:

Melt the butter over a medium heat and add a finely chopped shallot.

Cook for five or six minutes then add 1 tsp of white wine vinegar.

Cook for another couple of minutes then stir in yoghurt, mustard, capers and a small bunch of tarragon, chopped.

Reduce the heat and cook gently for two or three minutes until simmering, season then serve.

Spicy Chimichurri

Ingredients:

1 clove of garlic

1 red chilli

a small bunch each of coriander and parsley

3 tbsps. of red wine vinegar

2 tbsps. of olive oil

Method:

Put 1 clove of garlic, 1 red chilli, a small bunch each of coriander and parsley and 3 tbsps. of red wine vinegar in a small food processor.

Blitz until finely chopped then add 2 tbsps. of olive oil and blitz again.

Season and refrigerate until serving.

Chermoula

Ingredients:

1 large handful of cilantro (coriander) leaves, chopped

1 large handful of flat leaf parsley leaves, chopped

1 large handful of mint leaves, chopped

3 garlic cloves, chopped

2 tsps. ground cumin

2 tsps. ground coriander

1 tsp paprika

1 small red chilli, deseeded and chopped

3 tbsps. lemon juice

1/2 cup olive oil

freshly ground black pepper

Method:

Combine the herbs, garlic, spices, chilli and lemon juice in the bowl of a food processor.

With the motor running, drizzle in the oil and process until smooth. Season with salt and pepper.

The chermoula will last, stored in an airtight container, for 3—4 days in the fridge.

Great for chicken and fish and can be used as a marinade or sauce.

Red Capsicum Pesto

Ingredients:

2 red capsicums (peppers), halved and seeded

2 tbsps. olive oil

2 cloves garlic

50 g/1.7 oz parmesan

2 tbsps. pine nuts

Method:

Preheat oven to 180C (356F).

Place capsicums in a shallow baking dish skin-side up and drizzle with half the oil. Roast for 25 minutes. Remove from oven, cover with foil and allow to cool slightly. Peel off and discard skin.

Place all ingredients in a food processor and blend to a smooth paste. Season to taste.

Serve with grilled lamb, beef or chicken, or use to coat lamb fillets before barbecuing them.

Simple Capsicum Relish

Ingredients:

3 red capsicums (peppers), quartered, deseeded

1 tbsp. olive oil

1 small red onion, coarsely chopped

2 fresh rosemary sprigs, halved

1/3 cup red wine vinegar

1/3 cup, firmly packed brown sugar

Method:

Combine all ingredients and bring to the boil, reduce heat and simmer for 30 minutes, stirring occasionally.

Refrigerate overnight before serving.

Parsley relish

Ingredients:

1 bunch flat-leaf (Italian) parsley

6 anchovy fillets

2 tbsps. baby capers

grated zest of 2 lemons

1-1/2 cup lemon juice

1/4 cup olive oil

freshly ground black pepper

Method:

Place all ingredients except oil and pepper in a food processor. Lightly process, then, with the motor still running, add enough oil to form a thick paste. Season to taste with pepper.

Serve cooked lamb or beef with a dollop of relish on top.

Black Bean & Sesame Sauce

Ingredients:

half a can of drained and rinsed black beans

1 tsp of soft dark brown sugar

2 tsp of honey

1 tsp of Chinese five-spice powder

1/2 tsp of grated ginger

1 red chilli

2 tsp of tahini paste

2 tbsps. of cider vinegar

2 tsp of low sodium soy sauce

5 tbsps. of water

Method:

Put half a can of drained and rinsed black beans into a food processor. Add sugar, honey, Chinese five-spice powder, grated ginger, red chilli, tahini paste, cider vinegar, soy sauce and the water. Blend until very smooth then pour into a saucepan and bring to a simmer.

Cook for around five minutes or until glossy and thick, stirring all the time.

A very versatile sauce that can be used with most meats, stir fry, and even in salads.

Quick Red Wine Sauce

Ingredients:

2/3 cup beef stock

1/2 cup red wine

2 tsp of dark brown sugar

1 tsp of balsamic vinegar

Method:

Pour beef stock into a saucepan and reduce by half. Then add the red wine, sugar and balsamic vinegar.

Leave to cook for another 10 minutes over a high heat or until the sauce has reduced by half again.

Season to taste and serve.

Great with beef.

Mushroom Sauce

Ingredients:

1 tbsp. of olive oil

6 chestnut mushrooms, sliced

1 crushed garlic clove

2 tbsps. of brandy

4 tbsps. of double cream

1 tsp of wholegrain mustard

Method:

Pour olive oil into a saucepan over a high heat and add the mushrooms.

Fry for 5 minutes or until golden then stir in garlic, brandy and cook until the brandy has almost totally evaporated.

Then stir in the double cream and mustard. Reduce the heat and bring to a simmer.

Cook for two or three minutes more than season and serve.

Horseradish Cream Sauce

Ingredients:

1 cup sour cream

1/4 cup grated fresh horseradish

1 tbsp. Dijon mustard

1 tsp white wine vinegar

1/2 tsp kosher salt

1/4 tsp freshly ground black pepper

Method:

Place all of the ingredients into a medium mixing bowl and whisk until the mixture is smooth and creamy.

Place in the refrigerator for at least 4 hours or overnight to allow flavors to meld.

Sauce can be stored in the refrigerator in an airtight container for 2 to 3 weeks.

Garlic Wine Sauce

Ingredients:

3 tbsps. minced shallots

3 tbsps. minced garlic

1/2 tsp salt

4 turns freshly ground black pepper

1 1/2 cups veal stock or brown chicken stock

1/2 cup dry red wine

2 tbsps. unsalted butter, at room temperature

Method:

Combine the shallots, garlic, salt and pepper in a small nonreactive saucepan over high heat.

Stir in the stock and the wine and bring to a boil.

Cook over high heat for 15 minutes.

Swirl in the butter, remove from the heat, and continue to whisk in the butter until thoroughly incorporated.

Great with most meats especially roasts.

Apple, Onion and Cider Sauce

Ingredients:

2 to 3 tbsps. olive oil

1 large red onion, cut into large pieces

1 sweet cooking apple, cored and cut into large pieces

3 tbsps. apple cider vinegar

1 1/2 cups low-sodium chicken broth

2 tbsps. cold unsalted butter

1 handful fresh parsley, roughly chopped

Method:

Add the onion and apple to a frying pan along with 1 tbsp. oil and increase the heat to high.

Cook, tossing, until the onion has wilted slightly and the apple is golden brown, about 2 minutes.

Add the vinegar and use a wooden spoon to scrape the pan.

Let the mixture boil until the vinegar becomes syrupy, about 1 minute.

Add the chicken broth and return to a boil.

Cook until the broth reduces by half. Remove from the heat, season with pepper and whisk in the butter.

Great with Chicken and Pork.

Tangy Mustard Sauce

Ingredients:

2 tsps. olive oil

2 minced garlic cloves

1/4 cup dry white wine

1/4 cup chicken broth

2 tbsps. maple syrup

2 tbsps. Dijon mustard

3/4 tsp chopped fresh rosemary

1/2 tsp freshly ground black pepper

Method:

Heat olive oil in a skillet over medium heat.

Add minced garlic to pan; sauté 30 seconds, stirring constantly being careful not to discolour.

Stir in wine, chicken broth, maple syrup, and mustard and bring to a boil.

Cook until reduced to 1/4 cup (about 5 minutes), stirring occasionally.

Stir in rosemary and black pepper.

Spicy Orange Sauce

Ingredients:

1 tbsp. grated ginger

2/3 cup chicken broth or low-sodium chicken stock

3 tbsps. orange marmalade

1 1/2 tbsps. low-sodium soy sauce

1 1/2 tsps. fresh lemon juice

3/4 tsp hot chili sauce

Method:

Heat a skillet over medium-high heat and add a little oil.

Add grated ginger and sauté for 1 minute, stirring constantly.

Stir in chicken broth, orange marmalade, and soy sauce and bring to a boil.

Cook until mixture is slightly thick. Stir in fresh lemon juice and chili sauce.

Mango Salsa

Ingredients:

1 large mango, peeled and diced

1/2 cup peeled, diced cucumber

1/2 cup diced capsicum (bell pepper)

1 tbsp. finely chopped jalapeno (optional)

1/3 cup diced red onion

1 tbsp. lime juice

1/3 cup roughly chopped cilantro leaves

pepper

Method:

Combine the mango, cucumber, capsicum, jalapeno, red onion, lime juice and cilantro leaves and mix well. Season with pepper to taste.

Some people love the fresh crisp capsicum (bell pepper) if not, you can saute to soften and allowing to cool, or omit.

Great with white meats.

Warm Citrus Dressing

Ingredients:

1 tbsp. marmalade

1 tbsp. Dijon mustard

2 tbsp. red wine vinegar

1 tbsp. finely grated orange rind

2 oranges

2 tbsp. extra virgin olive oil

Freshly cracked pepper

Method:

Combine reserved mustard, marmalade, vinegar and orange rind in a saucepan and heat through. Remove from heat. Add olive oil, season with salt and pepper to taste. Remove rind and pith from oranges and segment into pieces.

Great with BBQ pork.

Tarragon Sauce

Ingredients:

2 tbsps. olive oil

1/2 cup mayonnaise

2 tbsps. Dijon mustard

2 tbsps. olive oil

4 cloves garlic, minced

1 tbsp. lemon juice

1 tbsp. finely grated lemon zest

2 tbsps. chopped fresh tarragon (or 2 tsp dried)

1/4 tsp ground black pepper

Method:

Whisk together the mayonnaise, mustard, olive oil, garlic, lemon juice, tarragon, and pepper

Great with Chicken.

Lemon-Herb Butter Sauce

Ingredients:

2 tbsps. finely chopped shallots (scallions/spring onions)

1/4 cup dry white wine

3 tbsps. fresh lemon juice

6 tbsps. butter (chilled)

1 tbsp. chopped fresh dill

1 tbsp. finely chopped fresh chives

1/8 tsp pepper

Method:

In small saucepan, combine shallots, wine and 3 tbsps. lemon juice.

Bring to a boil over medium-high heat.

Reduce heat to medium and cook for 5 to 7 minutes, stirring occasionally.

Remove from heat.

Stir in cold butter 1 tbsp. at a time until each is well blended. Stir in dill, chives and pepper.

Great with fish and chicken.

Grilled Salmon Sauce

Ingredients:

2 tbsps. butter

2 tbsps. brown sugar

2 garlic cloves, minced

1 tbsp. lemon juice

2 tsp soy sauce

1/2 tsp pepper

1/2 tsp minced fresh ginger (or ginger powder)

Method:

In a small saucepan, combine ingredients. Cook and stir until sugar is dissolved.

Brush on salmon while grilling.

Apple Sauce

Approx. 4 servings.

Ingredients:

1/2 cup unsalted butter

5 Granny Smith apples

1/2 cup brown sugar

1/2 cup raisins

1/4 cup apple juice

Method:

Peel, core and slice apples.

Melt butter in a pan. Add apples and stir to coat apple slices with butter.

Sprinkle brown sugar over apple slices and toss to coat.

Add apple juice and raisins. Bring to a boil then reduce heat and simmer for 10-15 minutes. Mash with a fork or potato masher.

Great with pork.

Roast Meat Gravy

Ingredients:

30 g/1 oz butter

1/2 large onion, chopped finely

1 clove garlic, chopped

1/2 tsp dried thyme

1 1/2 tbsp. plain flour

1 1/2 cup chicken stock

Method:

Cook onion, garlic and thyme for 5 mins over medium heat, until the onion softens, add flour and combine, leave it on the heat for another minute, then add the stock, mixing constantly to avoid any lumps.

Allow it thicken, stirring constantly. Add pepper to taste.

If it thickens up too much, simply add a little hot water, and mix.

Great with any roast meat.

Herb Sauce

Ingredients:

1 tsp black pepper

2 tsps. garlic powder

1/2 tsps. celery salt

1 tsp celery seeds

2-1/2 tsps. dry mustard

2 tsps. paprika

Method:

Mix all ingredients and store in an airtight container.

To prepare sauce for one portion of meat, melt 1 tbsp. unsalted butter or olive oil and add 1/2 tbsp. of herb sauce mix.

Pour over meat and bake in the oven or use as a sauce topping on chicken, fish or pork.

Cranberry Sauce

Ingredients:

12 oz/340 g of fresh or frozen cranberries

1 cup sugar

1 strip orange or lemon zest

2 tbsps. water

Method:

Add cranberries to a saucepan and saving 1/2 cup for later.

Add 1 cup sugar, 1 strip orange or lemon zest and 2 tbsps. water to the pan and cook over low heat, stirring occasionally, until the sugar dissolves and the cranberries are soft, about 10 minutes.

Increase the heat to medium and cook until the cranberries burst, about 12 minutes.

Reduce the heat to low and stir in the reserved cranberries.

Cool to room temperature before serving.

Endless uses. Great for poultry and pork, but can also be used in desserts.

Salsa Verde

Ingredients:

1 egg

1 bunch curly-leaf parsley, leaves picked

1 bunch mint, leaves picked

2 tbsps. drained capers

2-1/2 tbsps. chopped gherkins

4 anchovy fillets, drained of oil and coarsely chopped

2-1/2 tbsps. lemon juice

2 tsps. Dijon mustard

1 tbsp. olive oil

approximately 150 ml/5 fl oz salt-reduced vegetable stock

Method:

Hard-boil the egg in a small saucepan of simmering water for 7-8 minutes, then drain well and cool in cold water. Peel and set aside.

Place the remaining ingredients in a food processor. Chop the egg and add to the mixture, then process until a coarse paste forms, adding more stock or water if necessary. Season to taste, then serve.

Very universal sauce. Can be used as a dipping sauce or with any meat and most veg.

Salsa Verde (Egg-less)

Ingredients:

a small bunch of parsley

a small bunch of chives

a small bunch of mint

1 tsp of capers

two or three chopped anchovies

a crushed clove of garlic

juice of one lemon

3 tbsps. of olive oil

Method:

Chop a small bunch each of parsley, chives and mint into small pieces and mix in a bowl with 1 tsp of capers, two or three chopped anchovies, a crushed clove of garlic, the juice of one lemon and 3 tbsps. of olive oil. Mix it well and season to taste.

Very universal sauce. Can be used as a dipping sauce or with any meat and most veg.

Onion and Red Wine Puree

Ingredients:

1 tbsp. olive oil

4 sprigs thyme

4 onions, thinly sliced

1 1/2 tbsps. red wine vinegar

1/2 cup red wine

1 cup salt-reduced chicken or vegetable stock

Method:

Heat the oil in a saucepan over medium heat, then add the thyme and onion. Reduce the heat to low-medium, then cover and cook, stirring often, for 20 minutes or until the onion is very tender.

Add the remaining ingredients and stir to combine, then bring to simmering point. Cook over low heat, stirring occasionally, for about 20 minutes or until the liquid has reduced. Remove the thyme and discard.

Transfer the mixture to a food processor then process until smooth. Return to the saucepan and cook, stirring, over medium heat for 3-4 minutes to reheat, then serve.

Great for beef.

Olive Gremolata

Ingredients:

1 bunch flat-leaf (Italian) parsley

grated zest of 1 lemon

juice of 1/2 lemon

2 cloves garlic

100 g/3.5 oz pitted green olives

1/4 cup olive oil

freshly ground black pepper

Method:

Place all ingredients except the oil and pepper in a food processor. Lightly process, then, with the motor still running, add enough oil to form a thick paste. Season to taste with pepper.

Serve on top of baked fish or chicken.

Coriander Gremolata

Ingredients:

1 tbsp. olive oil
zest of 2 lemons, finely chopped
1 tsp crushed garlic
1/4 cup chopped coriander (cilantro)

Method:
Mix all the ingredients until well combined. Use topping on soups and salads or in summery pasta dishes.

Very universal.

Yoghurt sauce

Ingredients:

1 cup greek yoghurt

1 tbsp. chopped mint

1/2 clove garlic, finely chopped

2 tsps. lemon juice

1/2 tsp ground cumin

Method:

Place all ingredients in a bowl and mix well. Season to taste. Cover and refrigerate for 10 minutes before using. If the sauce is too thick, add a little water to thin it out.

Serve with grilled lamb or chicken.

Miso Sesame Sauce

Ingredients:

2 tbsps. sesame seeds

1 tbsp. red miso paste

1 tsp brown sugar

1 tsp grated ginger

1 tbsp. lemon juice

1/2 cup low-sodium chicken stock or chicken bone broth

Method:

Fry sesame seeds in a dry non-stick frying pan over medium heat for 5 minutes, or until golden.

Place all ingredients in a bowl and mix well. Serve drizzled over fish, chicken or vegetables.

Homemade No Salt Tomato sauce

Ingredients:
80 g Butter
80 g Bacon pieces, rough cut
80 g Onions, cut into small pieces
80 g Carrots, cut into small pieces
80 g Celery, cut into small pieces
100 g Flour
150 g Tomato paste
Garlic 1 clove
4 Peppercorns
1.1 L White stock
10 g Sugar
Bay leaf piece
Thyme sprig

Method:
Melt the butter in a large stewpan, add the bacon pieces and fry off lightly.

Add the onions, carrots and celery and fry to take some colour.

Cool for 2 minutes and add the flour.

Return to a moderate heat and cook, stirring until a fawn colour is achieved.

Add the tomato paste and stir well.

Add the stock gradually, stirring until it boils.

Add the garlic, bay leaf, thyme, and sugar and simmer for 1 hour. Stir frequently to avoid burning on the bottom of the pan.

Add pepper as desired and pass through a fine strainer.

Mint Sauce

Ingredients:
2 tsp Mint, fresh
2 tsp Castor sugar
1/3 cup Vinegar

Method:
Wash and drain the mint and pick it over.

Place on a board with the sugar and chop together (so that the sugar takes up the juice from the mint leaves).

Add to the vinegar.

Hoisin Sauce

Ingredients:
juice of 1 orange

2 tbsps. almond butter or tahini

1 tsp grated garlic

1 tbsp. grated ginger

2 tsps. apple cider vinegar

2 tsps. honey

4 tbsps. tamari

1/2 tsp Chinese five spice powder

1 1/2 tsps. sesame oil

1/2 tsp dried chilli flakes or powder

2 tsps. tomato paste

2 tbsps. water

Method:
Place all the ingredients in a saucepan and bring to a simmer over medium-low heat.

Cook for 5 minutes, stirring constantly. Allow to cool.

Transfer the sauce to a blender and blend until smooth.

Store in a glass jar in the fridge for up to 2 weeks.

Worcestershire Sauce

Ingredients:

1/2 cup apple cider vinegar

2 1/2 tbsps. tamari

1/2 tsp ground ginger

1/2 tsp mustard powder

1/2 tsp onion powder

1/2 tsp garlic powder

1/4 tsp ground cinnamon

1/4 tsp freshly ground black pepper

Method:

Combine all the ingredients with 2 tbsps. of water in a saucepan and bring to the boil over medium heat, stirring occasionally.

Reduce the heat to low and simmer for 10 minutes.

Remove from the heat and allow to cool.

Pour into a sterilised bottle and store in the fridge for up to 1 month.

Yellow Curry Paste

Ingredients:
6 dried long red chillies, soaked in hot water for 30 minutes

4 tbsps. coconut oil

10 garlic cloves, finely chopped

6 red Asian shallots, finely chopped

1 tsp shrimp paste

5 cm piece or ginger, grated

25 cm piece of galangal or ginger, grated

5 cm piece of fresh turmeric, grated (or 2 tablespoons ground turmeric)

4 kaffir lime leaves, chopped

1 tsp sea salt

Method:
Drain the chillies reserving 4 tbsps. of the soaking liquid.

Melt the oil in a frying pan over medium heat. Add the chillies and the remaining ingredients and cook, stirring occasionally, for 5—10 minutes until softened and fragrant.

Transfer the chilli mixture to the bowl of a food processor, add the reserved soaking liquid and blend to a smooth paste.

Store in a sealed container in the refrigerator for up to 1 month.

Artichoke Hummus

Ingredients:
1 x 425 g (15 oz) Can Chickpeas (garbanzo beans) or 3/4 cup dried chickpeas, cooked

1 x 400 g (14 oz) can Artichoke hearts in water

2 garlic, peeled

3 tbsps. tahini

1 tbsp. olive oil

juice of 1 medium lemon

1 tsp ground cumin. lightly roasted

freshly ground black pepper, to taste

Method:
Drain the chickpeas, reserving the liquid.

Drain the artichokes and squeeze them to get rid of the excess water inside them

Add all the ingredients, except the reserved chickpea liquid, to a food processor and blend until smooth. If the mixture is too thick, add some of the reserved liquid.

Season with salt and pepper to taste and serve.

Mushroom-Onion Gravy

Ingredients:

1 tbsp. olive oil

1 yellow onion, diced

1 clove garlic

1 cup sliced mushrooms

1 tbsp. whole wheat flour

1 1/2 cups water

1 1/2 tbsps. powdered vegetable broth

2 1/2 tbsps. flax oil

Method:

Heat olive oil and sauté onions and garlic until softened.

Add mushrooms and sauté 2-3 min.

Stir in flour and continue to sauté for 1 min.

Slowly add water with whisk until smooth.

Add broth and cook, allowing sauce to thicken.

Remove from heat and allow to cool.

Add flax oil and serve.

Simple Honey Mustard Sauce

Ingredients:

1/2 cup mayonnaise

2 tbsps. Dijon mustard

2 tbsps. honey

Method:

Stir all ingredients together.

Sour Cream Dill Sauce

Ingredients:

225 g/8 oz Sour cream (could sub with greek yoghurt)

2 tbsps. Fresh dill, chopped

2 tbsps. Fresh lemon juice

1 clove Garlic, minced

Method:

Mix ingredients together in a food processor or blender until smooth.

Refrigerate overnight.

Serve over seafood or fresh vegetables.

Homemade Soy Sauce

Ingredients:

1½ cups low sodium beef stock or chicken bone broth

3 tsp balsamic vinegar

2 tsp molasses

1/4 tsp ground ginger

1 pinch white pepper

1 pinch garlic powder

1 pinch onion powder

Method:

In a saucepan over medium heat, stir together all of the ingredients and bring to a boil.

Continue to boil gently until liquid is reduced to about 1 cup, for about 15 minutes.

Store in an airtight container, refrigerated, for up to one week.

Teriyaki Sauce

Ingredients:

5 tbsps. of low salt or homemade soy sauce

3 tbsps. of sake

2 tbsps. of mirin

1/2 tsp of ginger, grated

1 tsp of honey

1 sliced spring onion

Method:

Mixing together soy sauce, sake, mirin, ginger and honey.

Pour the mix into a small saucepan and bring to a simmer and cook for around five minutes or until slightly thickened.

Remove from the heat and stir in 1 sliced spring onion.

Serve

Lime Ginger Sauce

Ingredients:

1 cup White grape juice

1/4 cup Fresh lime juice

1/3 cup White wine vinegar

1 tbsp. Minced fresh ginger

1 tbsp. Minced fresh garlic

1/2 cup Heavy cream

1 1/2 sticks Cold unsalted butter, cut into chunks

1/4 cup Thai sweet chili sauce

Method:

In a heavy saucepan over medium heat, combine grape juice, lime juice, vinegar, ginger and garlic.

Bring to a boil; reduce by 90 percent to a light syrup.

Add cream and reduce by 60 percent, stirring carefully so as not to scorch the sauce.

Reduce heat to low and gradually stir in the cold butter chunks.

Stir in chili sauce.

Season with pepper.

Reserve and keep warm. Great for seafood and white meats.

BBQ Sauce

Ingredients:

1/4 cup Low-sodium Worcestershire sauce

1/4 cup Low-sodium or homemade soy sauce

1/4 cup White vinegar

2 tbsps. Canola oil

2 tbsps. Mustard

3/4 cup low salt ketchup/homemade tomato sauce

1/2 tsp Garlic powder

1/2 tsp Onion powder

1/8 tsp Ground black pepper

Method:

Use a whisk or processor to blend all ingredients well.

Garlic Rosemary Sauce

Ingredients:

2 garlic cloves, chopped

freshly ground black pepper

2 tbsps. olive oil

2 tbsps. rosemary

2 tbsps. fresh lemon juice

1/2 cup chicken stock

1 tbsp. butter

Method:

Add garlic, rosemary, lemon juice, and stock to skillet and over high heat, stirring for 1 minute.

Whisk in butter.

Great for lamb.

Almond Herb Pesto

Ingredients:
1 small bunch chives

1 small bunch flat-leaf (Italian) parsley

1 small bunch basil

1 small bunch coriander (cilantro)

1 cup almonds

2 large cloves garlic

2 tsps. herb salt

1/2 cup olive oil

Juice of 1 lemon

Method:
Add all the ingredients to a blender or food processor and pulse until coarsely blended.

Store in an airtight container in the refrigerator for up to 5 days.

Beef or Lamb Sauce

Ingredients:

1/2 cup red wine

1 tbsp. balsamic vinegar

1 tbsp. olive oil

sprigs of thyme

sprigs of rosemary

1 clove of garlic, crushed

2 bay leaves

2 spring onions (scallions), roughly chopped

Add all ingredients together and stir to mix. Drizzle over cooked meats or use as marinade or baste.

Ginger Soy

Ingredients:

1/4 cup soy sauce

1 tsp grated ginger

2 tsps. honey

1 tbsp. lemon juice

Add all ingredients together and stir to mix.

Can be used for dipping, with noodles, or with vegetables as desired.

Seafood Sauce

Ingredients:

1 tbsp. olive oil

2 tbsps. white wine vinegar

2 tsps. ground fennel

1/2 clove garlic, finely chopped

Add all ingredients together and stir to mix. Great for drizzling over seafood or dipping.

Chilli and Lime Seafood Sauce

Ingredients:

1 tsp sugar

1/3 cup light soy sauce

juice of 2 limes

1 tsp fish sauce

1/2 red chilli, finely sliced

1 tsp sesame oil

1 clove garlic, crushed

1 x thumb size piece ginger, shredded

3 spring onions (scallions), finely sliced

Add all ingredients together and stir to mix. Great for seafood.

Thai Sauce

Ingredients:

1/4 cup lime juice

2 tbsps. fish sauce

1 small red chilli, finely chopped

1 tsp brown sugar

1/4 cup coriander (cilantro) leaves

Add all ingredients together and stir to mix. Can be used as a dipping sauce as desired..

Marinades, Rubs and Spice Blends

Coriander Marinade

Ingredients:

2 tbsp. finely chopped coriander root and stem

1 tbsp. freshly grated ginger

1 tbsp. chilli paste

1 1/2 tbsp. fish sauce

1 tbsp. fresh lime juice

1/2 tbsp. brown sugar

Method:

Combine coriander root and stem, ginger and chilli and rub into Pork. Stir to combine fish sauce, lime juice and brown sugar.

Great for pork.

Maple Syrup Marinade

Ingredients:

1/3 cup maple syrup

1 1/2 tbsp. Dijon mustard

1 tbsp. vegetable oil

Freshly cracked pepper

Method:

Combine maple syrup, mustard, oil and pepper in a large flat container.

Great for pork.

Chinese Five Spice Marinade

Ingredients:

2 tbsp. soy sauce

1/2 tbsp. Chinese five spice

2 tbsp. peanut oil

Method:

Combine ingredients.

Great for pork.

Orange and Chilli Marinade

Ingredients:

2 tbsp. finely grated orange rind

1/4 cup fresh orange juice

1 tbsp. red chilli paste

1 tbsp. finely grated ginger

Method:

Combine ingredients in a non-metallic bowl and add Pork. Cover and chill for 30 minutes, turning once.

Great for pork.

Plum and Soy Marinade

Ingredients:

1 cup plum sauce

1/2 cup low-sodium soy sauce

Method:

Combine the plum sauce and soy sauce in a small bowl and mix well.

Great for pork.

Lemon Mustard Marinade

Ingredients:

Juice and rind of 1 lemon

1 tbsp. olive oil

1 tbsp. Dijon mustard

1 tbsp. parsley, chopped

1 cup apple sauce for serving

Method:

Combine the lemon juice and rind, olive oil, mustard and parsley in a glass bowl and mix well.

Great for pork.

Turkish Spice Blend

Ingredients:

1/3 cup ground cumin

3 tbsps. dried mint

3 tbsps. dried oregano

2 tbsps. paprika

2 tbsps. freshly ground black pepper

2 tsps. hot paprika

Method:

Combine all the ingredients in a bowl and mix well. Store in an airtight container in the pantry for up to 3 months.

Baharat

Ingredients:
4 parts paprika
4 parts ground black pepper
1 part ground coriander
1 part ground cloves
1 part ground cardamom
1 part ground cumin
1 part ground cinnamon
1 part ground ginger
1 part ground dried chilli
1/2 part ground allspice

Blend together and store in an airtight jar. Can be used as a dry rub for grilled meats or as an ingredient in other recipes.

The Dish Seasoning

Ingredients:

1/2 tsp paprika

1 tbsp. garlic powder

1 tsp basil

1 tsp marjoram

1 tsp thyme

1 tsp parsley

1 tsp rosemary

1 tsp ginger powder

1 tsp onion powder

1 tsp sage

1 tsp black pepper

Method:

Mix well and store in an airtight jar. A very universal seasoning, use anywhere!

Mustard and Herb Rub

Ingredients:

2 tbsp. Dijon mustard

1 tbsp. finely chopped flat leaf parsley

2 tbsp. finely chopped mint

2 tbsp. finely chopped chives

Freshly cracked black pepper

Method:

Combine mustard, herbs and pepper and spread evenly over both sides of the Pork. Pan-fry or BBQ Pork as usual. Avoid high heat which may burn coating.

Cumin and Coriander Rub

Ingredients:

1 tbsp. ground cumin

1 tbsp. ground coriander

1 tbsp. sweet ground paprika

1 1/2 tbsp. finely cracked black pepper

Method:

Place Pork steaks onto a plate. Combine cumin, coriander, paprika, pepper and salt in a bowl and stir well. Sprinkle and gently rub spices into Pork, coating both sides. BBQ or pan-fry Pork as usual.

Pepper Rub

Ingredients:

2 tbsp. sweet paprika

1 tbsp. cracked black pepper

1 tbsp. finely grated fresh ginger

1/2 tbsp. ground sage

Method:

Combine paprika, pepper, ginger, salt and sage.

Lightly rub this seasoning over both sides of the Pork.

BBQ or pan-fry Pork as usual.

Greek Rub

Ingredients:

1/4 cup lemon juice

2 tsps. lemon zest

1 tbsp. chopped flat-leaf (Italian) parsley

1 tbsp. chopped basil

1 clove garlic, finely chopped

2 tbsps. olive oil

2 tsps. Oregano

Add all ingredients together and stir to mix. Can be used for flavouring meats as beef and lamb.

Tandoori Rub

Ingredients:

1/3 cup tandoori paste

1 tsp ground cumin

1 tbsp. lemon juice

250 g reduced-fat natural yoghurt

1 clove garlic, crushed

Add all ingredients together and stir to mix. Can be used for flavouring meats as Chicken beef and lamb.

Five-Spice Chinese Rub

Ingredients:

2 tbsps. oyster sauce

1 tbsp. hoi sin sauce

1 tbsp. dry sherry

1/2 clove garlic, crushed

1 tsp five-spice powder

Add all ingredients together and stir to mix. Can be used for flavouring meats as pork.

Desserts

Coconut Berry Jelly

Ingredients:

1 cup (250ml/9 fl oz) of coconut milk
2 teaspoons of powdered gelatine
1/2 teaspoon of natural vanilla essence
1/2 cup of sugar
¼ cup of fresh berries (strawberry/blueberry/raspberry as you desire, thaw if frozen)

Method:

Chop the fruit into smaller chunks and place into serving glass.

Add the sugar and gelatine to a small saucepan along with half of the milk. Heat on a low until the gelatine and sugar dissolves while stirring, add the rest of the milk and mix well. Allow to cool slightly then pour over the fruit and refrigerate until set.

Buttermilk Puddings with Fresh Berries

Ingredients:

1 vanilla bean, split

600 ml/20.2 fl oz buttermilk

7 tsps. powdered gelatine

1/4 cup (40 g/1.4 oz) sugar

250 ml/8.4 fl oz reduced-fat vanilla yoghurt

600 g/21 oz fresh seasonal berries (strawberries, raspberries, blueberries, etc.)

Method:

Add half the buttermilk and vanilla bean to a small saucepan and bring to a simmer. Remove from heat and sprinkle in gelatine while stirring to dissolve. Allow to cool slightly, stir in sugar, then strain through a fine-mesh sieve.

Combine the remaining buttermilk, yogurt, and gelatine mixture. Stir gently, then pour into 6 small ramekins or glasses. Refrigerate until set, about 2 hours.

Serve with the fresh berries.

Coconut-Sago Pudding with Mango

Ingredients:

1/3 cup (65 g/2.3 oz) sago

1/3 cup (75 g/2.6 oz) sugar

1 cup (250 ml/8.4 fl oz) Coconut Milk

1 mango, peeled and cut into small squares

Method:

Soak the sago in cold water to cover for 1 hour, then drain well. Combine the drained sago and 2 cups (500 ml/17 fl oz) water in a saucepan and slowly bring to simmering point. Cook the mixture, stirring often, over low-medium heat for 15 minutes or until the sago is translucent. Strain and rinse, set aside.

In a saucepan add the milk and sugar and stir over a low heat, add the sago, stirring again.

Serve warm or at room temperature with the mango.

Baked Apples

Ingredients:
2 Apples, large (Granny Smith)
20 g/.7 oz Seeded raisins (or sultanas)
40 g/1.4 oz (2 tbsps.) Brown sugar
pinch of Cinnamon
10 g/.35 oz Butter

Method:
Core the apples and make a circular cut in the skin around the equator.

Put the apples in a baking dish. Half fill the core hole with raisins, add sugar and the rest of the raisins. Put 5 g butter on top of each apple.

Pour just enough water in the baking dish to cover the surface.

Bake at 180C (356F) for about 40 minutes, until the apples are tender.

Serve with hot custard sauce.

Strawberry Smoothie

Ingredients:

2 cups of frozen strawberries

1 cup of yoghurt

1 cup of skimmed milk or soy milk

2 tbsp. of flax oil

Method:

Blend and serve! Garnish with a sprig of fresh mint.

Blueberry–Chia Seed Jam

Ingredients

3 cups fresh (or frozen and thawed) blueberries

2 teaspoons grated lemon zest

¼ cup fresh lemon juice

3 tablespoons (or more) pure maple syrup

¼ cup chia seeds

Method

Bring lemon zest, lemon juice, blueberries, and maple syrup to a simmer in a saucepan over medium heat and cook for 5 minutes, stirring occasionally.

Increase the heat and bring to a boil. Continue to cook, stirring occasionally for 5-10 minutes.

Stir in chia seeds and continue to cook for 1 minute. Remove from heat and allow the jam to cool and then add to heatproof jars. Cover and let cool completely. Chill until needed.

Pineberry-Chia Smoothie

Ingredients

1 cup Strawberries, ends removed, frozen

½ cup frozen pineapple chunks

¼ cup Blueberry–Chia Seed Jam

1 cup coconut water or unsweetened almond milk

1 tablespoon golden flaxseed oil (optional)

Method

Blend strawberry, pineapple, jam, coconut water, and oil in a blender until smooth.

Makes about 2 cups.

Made in the USA
Las Vegas, NV
04 May 2021